Genetic Aspects of
Speech and Language Disorders

Contributors

BARTON CHILDS

JUDITH A. COOPER

J. C. DeFRIES

ROSWELL ELDRIDGE

REBECCA FELTON

JOAN M. FINUCCI

ALBERT M. GALABURDA

NORMAN GESCHWIND

KENNETH K. KIDD

WILLIAM J. KIMBERLING

H. A. LUBS

CHRISTY L. LUDLOW

E. DAVID MELLITS

C. NETLEY

DAVID L. PAULS

B. F. PENNINGTON

ROBERT PLOMIN

PAUL SATZ

S. D. SMITH

RACHEL E. STARK

PAULA TALLAL

FRANK WOOD

JOSEF ZAIDE

Genetic Aspects of Speech and Language Disorders

Edited by

CHRISTY L. LUDLOW
JUDITH A. COOPER

Communicative Disorders Program
National Institute of Neurological and
Communicative Disorders and Stroke
Bethesda, Maryland

ACADEMIC PRESS   1983

A Subsidiary of Harcourt Brace Jovanovich, Publishers

New York   London
Paris   San Diego   San Francisco   São Paulo   Sydney   Tokyo   Toronto

ACADEMIC PRESS, INC.
111 Fifth Avenue, New York, New York 10003

United Kingdom Edition published by
ACADEMIC PRESS, INC. (LONDON) LTD.
24/28 Oval Road, London NW1   7DX

Library of Congress Cataloging in Publication Data
Main entry under title:

Genetic aspects of speech and language disorders.

  Bibliography: p.
  Includes index.
  1. Speech, Disorders of--Genetic aspects. 2. Lan-
guage disorders--Genetic aspects. I. Ludlow, Christy L.
II. Cooper, Judith A.
RC423.G45 1983   616.85'5042   83-10014
ISBN 0-12-459350-X

PRINTED IN THE UNITED STATES OF AMERICA

83 84 85 86   9 8 7 6 5 4 3 2 1

Contents

I

Introduction

1

Genetic Aspects of Speech and Language Disorders: Current Status and Future Directions

CHRISTY L. LUDLOW and JUDITH A. COOPER

2

Genetics: Fate, Chance, and Environmental Control

NORMAN GESCHWIND

II

Defining the Phenotype

3

Behavioral Attributes of Speech and Language Disorders

RACHEL E. STARK, E. DAVID MELLITS, and PAULA TALLAL

4

Physiological Specification of the Phenotype
in Genetic Language Disorders:
Prospects for the Use of Indicators
of Localized Brain Metabolism

FRANK WOOD and REBECCA FELTON

III

Investigation of Genotype:
Methodology and Research Designs

Contributors

Numbers in parentheses indicate the pages on which the authors' contributions begin.

BARTON CHILDS*(157)*, *Department of Pediatrics, Johns Hopkins University School of Medicine, Baltimore, Maryland 21205*

JUDITH A. COOPER*(3)*, *Communicative Disorders Program, National Institute of Neurological and Communicative Disorders and Stroke, Bethesda, Maryland 20205*

J. C. DeFRIES*(121)*, *Institute for Behavioral Genetics, University of Colorado, Boulder, Colorado 80309*

ROSWELL ELDRIDGE*(109)*, *Clinical Neurogenetic Studies, Neuroepidemiology Section, IRP, National Institute of Neurological and Communicative Disorders and Stroke, Bethesda, Maryland 20205*

REBECCA FELTON*(53)*, *Neuropsychology Section, Bowman Gray School of Medicine of Wake Forest University, Winston-Salem, North Carolina 27103*

JOAN M. FINUCCI*(157)*, *Department of Pediatrics, Johns Hopkins University School of Medicine, Baltimore, Maryland 21205*

ALBERT M. GALABURDA*(71)*, *Neurological Unit, Beth Israel Hospital, Boston, Massachusetts 02215*

NORMAN GESCHWIND*(21)*, *Department of Neurology, Harvard Medical School, Boston, Massachusetts 02215*

KENNETH K. KIDD*(197)*, *Department of Human Genetics, Yale University School of Medicine, New Haven, Connecticut 06510*

WILLIAM J. KIMBERLING*(151, 169)*, *Genetics Laboratory, Boys Town Institute for Communicative Disorders in Children, Omaha, Nebraska 68131*

H. A. LUBS*(169), Department of Genetics, University of Miami, Miami, Florida 33101*

CHRISTY L. LUDLOW*(3), Communicative Disorders Program, National Institute of Neurological and Communicative Disorders and Stroke, Bethesda, Maryland 20205*

E. DAVID MELLITS*(37), Department of Pediatrics, Johns Hopkins Hospital, Baltimore, Maryland 21205*

C. NETLEY*(179), Department of Psychology, Hospital for Sick Children, Toronto, Ontario, M5G 1X8, Canada*

DAVID L. PAULS*(139), Department of Human Genetics, Yale University School of Medicine, New Haven, Connecticut 06510*

B. F. PENNINGTON*(169), University of Colorado Medical Center, Denver, Colorado 80262*

ROBERT PLOMIN*(121), Institute of Behavioral Genetics, University of Colorado, Boulder, Colorado 80309*

PAUL SATZ*(85), Department of Psychiatry and Biobehavioral Sciences, University of California at Los Angeles School of Medicine, and Center for the Health Sciences, Los Angeles, California 90024*

S. D. SMITH*(169), Boys Town Institute for Communicative Disorders in Children, Omaha, Nebraska 68131*

RACHEL E. STARK*(37), Division of Hearing and Speech, John F. Kennedy Institute, Baltimore, Maryland 21205, and Department of Neurology, Johns Hopkins University School of Medicine, Baltimore, Maryland 21205*

PAULA TALLAL*(37), Department of Psychiatry, University of California at San Diego, La Jolla, California 92093*

FRANK WOOD*(53), Neuropsychology Section, Department of Neurology, Bowman Gray School of Medicine of Wake Forest University, Winston-Salem, North Carolina 27103*

JOSEF ZAIDE[1]*(85), Department of Psychology, University of Victoria, Victoria, British Columbia, V8W 2Y2 , Canada*

[1]Present address: Department of Psychology, Children's Hospital, Vancouver, British Columbia, V6H 3V4, Canada.

Preface

For many years, investigators have observed an apparent familial component to certain developmental speech and language disorders. However, the
etiological bases of those disorders have remained elusive, as have appropriate
methodologies for investigation. The recent emergence of the discipline of
behavioral genetics has altered the study of the hereditary bases of many behavioral traits, including specific cognitive abilities, psychopathology, and intelligence. The question naturally arises, does this discipline have the potential for
improving our understanding and treatment of speech and language disorders?

This book was organized to contribute to the answer. Part I, a review and
discussion of previous research and research needs, introduces the reader to
the current state of knowledge on this topic. Part II presents a description of
developmental and behavioral characteristics, or the phenotype, of speech- and
language-disordered individuals, including communication, sex, physiological,
and anatomical attributes. The focus of Part III is various methodological and
research designs that have been used or might be appropriate in investigation
of the genetic material, or genotype, responsible for language or learning deficits. Finally, Part IV presents current research relating genetics to specific communication and learning disorders, including dyslexia, sex chromosome abnormalities, and stuttering.

Genetic Aspects of Speech and Language Disorders provides to those
individuals with advanced training in speech and language disorders and/or
genetics a review of previous research, a discussion of current research and
available methodologies, and realistic directions for future research. It is hoped
that the ideas and information provided by the various contributors to this book
will give rise to innovative, productive investigations in this area.

In the fall of 1981, a group of individuals with established expertise in the fields of speech–language pathology, genetics, neurology, and psychology gathered to discuss issues and research related to the genetic aspects of speech and language disorders. Coming from a variety of backgrounds and training, these individuals nonetheless shared a common interest in attempting to blend the disciplines of behavioral genetics and communication disorders. Their task was to establish a base of knowledge about the area, to review genetic research methodologies with potential applicability to speech and language disorders, and to identify the most feasible and logical "first steps" for research. This book is one of the products of that gathering, but is far from a literal report of the presentations.

I

INTRODUCTION

1

Genetic Aspects of Speech and Language Disorders: Current Status and Future Directions

CHRISTY L. LUDLOW
JUDITH A. COOPER

The purpose of this book is to explore the possibilities of a genetic basis for some speech and language disorders. Little information is available regarding potential etiologies of primary developmental speech and language disorders, that is, those which do not occur in conjunction with other abnormalities, such as mental retardation, emotional disturbance, etc. For many years, it was thought that prenatal or perinatal brain injury could be responsible for developmental language disorders. However, studies of the birth histories of developmentally language-impaired children have not demonstrated a distinctive pre- or perinatal history of frank neurological insult (LaBenz & LaBenz, 1980). The National Collaborative Perinatal Project was the most extensive investigation of this question, and the results did not provide support for perinatal brain injury underlying these disorders (LaBenz & LaBenz, 1980). Similarly, Goldman (1979) has conducted studies in monkeys of the effects of prenatal cortical removals on subsequent adult learning behavior. Gross effects either during development or adulthood have not been found. Thus frank disturbances affecting brain development early in life cannot be assumed to underlie most developmental language disorders.

Other factors that have been proposed as contributing to the occurrence of these disorders include social, nutritional, and environmental factors. For many years the psychosocial factor was thought to be strong in disorders such as infantile autism and stuttering. However, families of children with these disorders do not have a greater frequency of poor language-learning environments or a higher familial incidence of mental illness. Thus the possibility of a neurological disorder that could have a genetic basis has been considered. In

3

ISBN 0-12-459350-X

infantile autism, the high proportion of other cognitive, sensory, and motoric disturbances accompanying the syndrome is a further indication that the behavioral components are probably not due to the environmental psychosocial abnormalities, and that autism is more likely the manifestation of a neurological disorder that could have a genetic basis (see Lockman, Swaiman, Drage, Nelson, & Marsden, 1979).

It has been proposed that stuttering behaviors may be learned (Brutten & Shoemaker, 1967; Johnson, 1944). However, the characteristics of this disorder have been found to be similar across cultures. This fact suggests that stuttering is not primarily a learned disorder since if this were the case one would expect cultural differences as in other socially learned behaviors. Further, a young child can develop stuttering when there is no other child in the community or social environment who stutters, suggesting that this disorder is most likely biologically based. In addition, the occurrence of abnormal patterns of timing and coordination of the oral and laryngeal musculature during speech have led several investigators to suggest that this disorder is a subtle disturbance of neuromotor control for speech (Freeman, 1979; Zimmerman, 1980). The possibility of genetic predisposing factors or defects contributing to the occurrence of such deviations during development cannot be disregarded.

The evidence for genetic predisposing factors in the occurrence of speech and language disorders, however, is indirect at best. Although there are instances of speech and language deficits occurring in association with genetic abnormalities (Kimberling & Brookhouser, 1981; Siegel-Sadewitz & Shprintzen, 1982) these are usually accompanied by other developmental abnormalities and the speech and/or language disorder is not the primary impairment and does not occur in every case (Lenneberg, 1964). Few, if any, developmental speech and language disorders have a well-documented chromosomal basis. Nonetheless, some studies do suggest a hereditary component to these disorders.

DELAYED SPEECH AND LANGUAGE DEVELOPMENT

The studies suggesting a hereditary component in the etiology of primary developmental language disorders have been descriptive case studies (Arnold, 1961; Luchsinger, 1970; Mattejat, Niebergall, & Nestler, 1980; Zaleski, 1966) with few exceptions, e.g., Mussafia (1964). There are methodological problems with most of these studies, bringing their interpretation into question. The criteria for selecting those with a language impairment are often unclear or absent. Terminology utilized in describing speech and language deficits may not be defined, or documented with formalized testing. Subject acquisition procedures are often questionable as are the methods used to determine whether a positive family history for the disorder is significant. Often parental reports of development of language, such as age at first word, must rely on memories of events

20–40 years in the past. Such procedures render the results open to bias and of questionable validity.

Some studies have examined the karyotpes[1] of speech- and language-delayed children. Garvey and Mutton (1973) studied 9 children with normal language comprehension but grossly defective expressive speech. Sex chromosome abnormalities were found in three cases; two were mosaics (46 XY, 47 XYY and 46 XY, 47 XY) and one was 48 XXYY. Evidence of minor chromosomal variation was not found. However, the 9 cases studied were selected from a pool of 450 children with severe speech and language problems, and only these 9 met the authors' subject selection criterion of normal language comprehension with impaired speech expression. Thus the 9 subjects constitute a specific subtype and are not representative of most children with developmental speech and language problems. Mutton and Lea (1980) conducted chromosomal analyses of 88 individuals aged 7–16, described as having "severe speech and language disorders." Four boys were identified with anomalies: 47 XXY; 47 XYY: 48 XXYY: and a low-grade mosaicism with trisomy 21. The incidence of such anomalies was greater than would be expected in a normal population.

The possibility of such chromosomal deviations being present in a large proportion of speech- and language-impaired children seems unlikely. Further investigations have supported such a claim. Tuncbilek, Kurultay, and Belgin (1978) found no minor or major chromosomal abnormalities in a group of 21 patients described as having speech delay in the absence of mental retardation or hearing loss. Hier, Atkins and Perlo's (1980) findings were similarly negative. Therefore, with the exception of Garvey and Mutton (1973), and Mutton and Lea's follow-up study (1980) the data currently available suggest that sex chromosome aberrations are not an important cause of primary disorders in the development of speech and language.

Although relatively few children with primary developmental language disorders have sex chromosome anomalies, when children with such anomalies are studied many are found to have communication impairments. Klinefelter's syndrome is associated with the occurrence in males of two or more X chromosomes in addition to the Y chromosome. Delays in language and articulatory acquisition are reported in 40–75% of the cases studied (Annell, Gustavson, & Tenstam, 1970; Haka-Ikse, Steward, & Cripps, 1978; Nielsen & Sillesen, 1976; Nielsen, Sorenson, & Sorenson, 1981). These delays often necessitate speech and language therapy (Funderburk & Ferjo, 1978; Puck, Tennes, Frankenburg, Bryant, & Robinson, 1975). In addition, stuttering and academic difficulties have been reported (Annell et al., 1970; Haka-Ikse et al., 1978). Verbal IQ scores were lower than performance IQ in some studies (Nielson et al., 1981; Puck et al., 1975) but equivalent in others (Funderburk and Ferjo, 1978). Some communicative impairments, such as poor abstraction and limited expressive lan-

---

[1]See definitions of genetic terms in the Glossary (p. 215).

6   Christy L. Ludlow and Judith A. Cooper

guage, persist into adulthood in some individuals with Klinefelter's (Funderburk & Ferjo, 1978).

The syndrome of 47 XYY in males is often associated with antisocial and aggressive behavior, very tall stature, and mild mental retardation (Kaplan, 1976). Ratcliffe (1982) reported that 9 of 18 boys with 47 XYY exhibited delayed speech primarily of a dyspraxic nature, with normal language comprehension. At various centers, between one-third and one-half of patients with this syndrome exhibited these same communicative impairments (Ratcliffe, 1982). Delays in expressive language, including reduced sentence length, poor intelligibility, and omission of most consonant sounds, have also been reported (Haka-Ikse et al., 1978; Nielsen & Sillesen, 1976; Valentine, McClelland, & Sergovich, 1971).

Females with trisomy X (47 XXX) often appear normal and do not exhibit particular physical or psychological characteristics. Pennington, Puck, and Robinson (1980) found speech delays in their longitudinal study of 11 47 XXX girls from infancy to school age. The mean age at first word was 19.8 months (range: 12–40 months) with word combinations first occurring at 32 months (range 24–45 months). Similar delays in speech and language milestones and comprehension and production deficits have been reported, with incidence figures varying from 20 to 80% of the subjects studied (Haka-Ikse et al., 1978; Nielsen & Sillesen, 1976; Nielsen et al., 1981: Pennington et al., 1980; Tennes, Puck, Bryant, Frankenburg, & Robinson, 1975). Nonetheless, psychological testing results have failed to reveal a significant verbal–performance discrepancy (Pennington et al., 1980; Ratcliffe, 1982) with only one exception (Nielsen et al., 1981). Learning and academic problems have also been reported with this population (Haka-Ikse et al., 1978; Hier et al., 1980; Ratcliffe, 1982).

In contrast to other sex chromosome aberrations, Turner's syndrome is not associated with an increased risk of speech and language impairments. Turner's, characterized by a single X chromosome in females (XO), is associated with normal language acquisition and functioning, but impaired nonverbal performance (Hier et al., 1980; Nielsen & Sillesen, 1976). Thus, with this exception, the presence of sex chromosome abnormalities carries with it the increased possiblity of speech and language delay.

To date, no studies have focused specifically on the genetic bases of developmental speech misarticulations. Although some individuals with speech misarticulations may have been included in genetic studies of delayed or impaired language development (e.g., Arnold, 1961; Mutton & Lea, 1980), phonological or articulatory disorders have not received separate attention. McLaughlin and Kriegsman (1980) studied a family with Renpenning's syndrome, or nonspecific X-linked mental retardation. They documented developmental dyspraxia as a predominant feature of the mental retardation. Pedigree information suggested an X-linked pattern of transmission for the dyspraxia. Others have reported delayed articulatory development with speech substitutions and omissions rather than a dyspraxia in X-linked mental retardation (Howard-Peebles, Stoddard, & Mims, 1979).

FLUENCY DISORDERS

Considerable attention has been given to the genetic contribution to the disorders of stuttering; however, cluttering has been largely ignored. Cluttering, characterized by hurried speech, dysrhythmia, and poor articulation, has been claimed to have a strong hereditary component (Bradford, 1970; Weiss, 1964), although formalized investigations have yet to be undertaken. Of all communication disorders, stuttering has received the most attention regarding its relationship to heredity. The concept of stuttering as a genetic disorder has gained increased acceptance in recent years. Information regarding the role of heredity in stuttering is available from four types of studies: familial incidence, spontaneous recovery, twins, and parental disfluencies (Sheehan & Costley, 1977). Although there tends to be agreement regarding a strong link between positive family history and stuttering, caution must be exercised in the interpretation of much of this research because of certain methodological issues. These include inadequate description of the sampling method, family members' contact with the stutterer, and relationship of family members to the proband (see Sheehan & Costley, 1977, for complete discussion).

There is an increased risk of stuttering for relatives of a stutterer, perhaps three to four times higher than the general population, and the risk is further increased if one parent is also a stutterer (Andrews & Harris, 1964; Chakravartti, Roy, Rao, & Chakravartti, 1979; Ehrman & Parsons, 1976; Howie, 1981a; Kidd, Reich, & Kessler, 1973; Pauls & Kidd, 1982; Porfert & Rosenfield, 1978). Monozygotic twins, derived from a single fertilized ovum with the same genetic material, have a significantly greater incidence of concordance for stuttering than dizygotic twins, who are no more similar genetically than other siblings within a family (Howie, 1981b). There is a strong sex effect. Males are affected between three to four times more frequently than females (Andrews & Harris, 1964; Ehrman & Parson, 1976; Porfert & Rosenfield, 1978; Sheehan & Costley, 1977). In addition, the risk of stuttering among relatives of the female probands seems greater than the risk among relatives of the male probands (Andrews & Harris, 1964; Kidd et al., 1973). Thus, although females are affected less frequently than males, affected females may be more "genetically loaded" than affected males (Ehrman & Parsons, 1976). The highest risk therefore occurs among male relatives of female stutterers and the lowest among female relatives of male stutterers (Andrews & Harris, 1964). Kidd, Heimbuch, and Records (1981) suggest that for a female to become a stutterer, it may be necessary for her to excede the threshold required for a male. These sex differences may be explained by the genetic concept of sex limitation, when expression of the same genotype is different in males and females (Andrews & Harris, 1964).

The contribution of learning or imitation to the establishment of stuttering is recognized, but most investigators (e.g., Andrews & Harris, 1964; Chakravartti et al., 1979; Ehrman & Parson, 1976;Kidd et al., 1981) downplay its importance as a major contributing factor for the following reasons. Many parents who stuttered recovered prior to the birth of a proband (Kidd et al., 1981). There are reports of adopted children who stutter with no stuttering history in the adopted family (Bloodstein, 1961). In families of stutterers, the frequency of postproband stutterers is no greater than the frequency of preproband stutterers, that is, stutterers tend to be randomly distributed among the birthranks (Gladstein, Seider, & Kidd, 1981). Most siblings of stutterers are nonaffected (Chakravartti et al., 1979). A cautionary finding, however, is the report that in some monozygotic twins, only one of the pair is a stutterer, suggesting that genetic factors alone are not sufficient to produce stuttering (Howie, 1981a).

Despite strong evidence of a nonenvironmental basis for stuttering, a genetic explanation is not readily forthcoming. Kidd et al. (1973) have suggested that stuttering may involve a dominant gene with a single locus and two alleles. If an individual is homozygous for the normal allele, stuttering would not occur. If an individual is homozygous for the stuttering allele, stuttering would almost always occur. Heterozygosity would be associated with stuttering 25% of the time in males but only 4% of the time in females, and environmental factors would affect only those individuals with heterozygosity. In contrast, other investigators claim stuttering may be wholly polygenic or multifactorial. For example, Andrews and Harris (1964) suggest that stuttering may be transmitted similarly to stature and intelligence, and that no one gene is essential. Rather, the genetic basis is provided by a number of genes acting together, perhaps creating an underlying predisposition. Most investigators agree that the exact method of transmission has yet to be determined (Chakravartti et al., 1979; Howie, 1981a, 1981b; Kidd et al., 1981).

DYSLEXIA AND OTHER LEARNING DISABILITIES

The possible genetic basis of dyslexia has been considered since the early 1900s (see Hallgren, 1950, for a review). The few chromosomal analyses that have been done with dyslexics failed to reveal abnormalities (Hier et al., 1980). As in other disorders discussed, males tend to be affected more frequently than females (Hallgren, 1950; Zahalkova, Vrzal, & Kloboukova, 1972). However, the proportion of dyslexics among the siblings of male and female probands has not been found to differ (Zahalkova et al., 1972).

Investigators have assessed family history in dyslexia by means of questionnaire (Omenn & Weber, 1978; Silver, 1971; Singer, Stewart, & Pulaski, 1981). Such investigations have revealed the following:

1. An incidence of family history for learning disability or dyslexia ranges

from 30 to almost 90% of the families of dyslexics (Hallgren, 1950; Silver, 1971).

2. There are similarities between the disabilities of the family members (mother, father, and/or siblings) and those of the proband (Childs & Finuci, 1979; Cole, 1964; DeFries, Singer, Foch, & Lewitter, 1978; Omenn & Weber, 1978).

3. When compared with parents of nondyslexic children, parents of dyslexics were found to read less, watch more television, and make fewer attempts to teach their children to read prior to entering school (DeFries et al., 1978), and they report an impact of their deficits on their career choice (Singer et al., 1981).

Less frequently, formalized testing of siblings and/or parents has been employed (Childs & Finucci, 1979; Decker & DeFries, 1980; Zahalkova et al., 1972). Both parents and siblings of probands performed more poorly than parents and siblings of non-reading-disabled children, on reading and on other language-related tasks (Decker & DeFries, 1980; DeFries et al., 1978; McGlannan, 1968). Deficits in reading ability, oral reading, and auditory memory have also been reported (Foch, DeFries, McClearn, & Singer, 1977).

Although investigators have frequently documented the generation-to-generation transmission of this disorder, no one pattern or mode of transmission is capable of explaining the variety of pedigrees reported. Certain methodological problems, such as small sample size and ascertainment and diagnostic difficulties may contribute to problems in determining the mode of inheritance (Lewitter, DeFries, & Elston, 1980). It is generally accepted that dyslexia represents a genetically heterogeneous disorder, whose mode of inheritance may involve the presence of a single dominant gene highly associated with reading disabilities (Hallgren, 1950; Zakalkova et al., 1972). However, the autosomal dominant hypothesis has been rejected by some investigators (e.g., Foch et al., 1977), because mothers and sisters of probands exhibit fewer deficiencies than males. An alternative explanation of the genetic bases is some multigenic influence (Childs & Finucci, 1979; Decker & DeFries, 1981; Foch et al., 1977; Kimberling & Brookhouser, 1981; Lewitter et al., 1980; Omenn & Weber, 1978). As with stuttering, there may be partial sex limitation in learning disability and dyslexia, explaining why the gene is manifested less frequently in females (Zahalkova et al., 1972). McGlannan (1968) suggested that dyslexia may have a "dual etiology." That is, in some cases there may be an inherited anomaly which alone causes the learning disorder, while in other cases there may be vulnerability to potentially disruptive factors frequently present during development.

Identifying subtypes among learning-disabled subjects based on their patterns of impairment could allow for a more precise study of etiology (Kimberling & Brookhouser, 1981). For example, dyslexics have been subgrouped according to whether visual or auditory deficits are associated with the reading disability (Childs & Finucci, 1979; Decker & DeFries, 1980; Omenn & Weber, 1978).

AUTISM

Research on infantile autism has moved away from a search for environmental–psychological bases toward a neurological focus, with an interest in possible genetic bases for the disorder. Chromosomal analyses of autistic children have failed to reveal abnormalities (see Spence, 1976). Although there is usually a negative family history for autism, this does not negate the possibility of a genetic component. It is rare for autists to marry. In addition, if a disorder is uncommon, the rate in relatives will be low even when the disorder is highly heritable (Folstein & Rutter, 1977). Support for a genetic component includes the general finding of parents without mental illness, the low recurrence rate within the immediate family, and the altered sex ratio among affected individuals (Spence, 1976). An increased incidence, albeit small (2%), of autism has been found in siblings of autistic individuals. Although this figure appears low, it is 50 times that of the general population (Folstein & Rutter, 1977; Ross & Pelham, 1981).

Because of the low incidence in families, and the fact that the syndrome of infantile autism encompasses a variety of behaviors, some investigators have focused on a broader spectrum of disorders in attempting to address the issue of a genetic basis. It may be that the syndrome of infantile autism is not inherited. Rather, it may be one form of a group of linguistic–cognitive impairments (Folstein & Rutter, 1977). For example, parents, siblings, and twins of autists have an increased incidence or history of language or speech disorders (Bartak, Rutter, & Cox, 1975; Folstein & Rutter, 1977). August, Stewart, and Tsai (1981) investigated the range of possible expressions of autism in 41 autistic probands and their biological siblings on a battery of psychological and academic measures. Of the 71 siblings, 11 (15.5%) met at least one criterion for a cognitive disability, as did only 1 of the 38 controls (3%). Four of the 11 exhibited gross disturbances in language acquisition, with no evidence of speech or a failure to use speech in a socially appropriate manner. Nine of the 11 had an IQ of less than 80 with 7 receiving special education. There were no factors that distinguished families with only a proband affected from families with a proband and an affected sibling. These results suggest a common genetic influence with variability in mode of expression.

The genetic component in infantile autism was highlighted in a twin study by Folstein and Rutter (1977), who evaluated 10 dizygotic (DZ) twin pairs and 11 monzygotic (MZ) pairs, with at least one of each pair being autistic. In the DZ pairs, none were concordant for autism, and only one was concordant for a language-based cognitive disability. In MZ pairs, four were concordant for infantile autism, and nine were concordant for some kind of cognitive disability, usually language. Such differences in concordance between the two types of twins supports a hereditary influence.

Determining what might be the mode of inheritance, however, has been difficult, because of the low incidence of marriage or parenthood among autists. Infantile autism may represent a combination of brain damage and inherited cognitive abnormalities (Folstein & Rutter, 1977).

RESEARCH CONSIDERATIONS

As indicated in the preceding discussion, the proposition of a genetic basis does not preclude the possibility of there being various types of neurological abnormalities underlying some of these speech and language disorders. Rather, it means only that a genetic defect or factor may be responsible for the neurological abnormality. The speech and language disorders observed during development, such as stuttering or delayed language development, may be twice removed from the original abnormality. The original abnormality may be genetic, either as an abnormality in the genotype or as a disturbance in the genetic material received from the parents. Such genetic abnormalities may then be expressed during neurological development, perhaps, as has been suggested by Galaburda (see Chapter 4 of this volume) and others, as abnormal cell migration patterns during brain development resulting in either partial or abnormal development of certain structures. This neurological abnormality may then be expressed in deviant or impaired development of certain cognitive skills such as language. Thus there are several levels of expression that must take place between the original primary defect in the genetic material and the behavioral signs manifested during development.

Other aspects of the child's genotype may determine its response to the genetic defect during neurological development. In addition, the social, environmental, and nutritional factors will contribute to a child's behavioral development and the effect the neurological abnormality may have on speech and language development.

These possible interactions among genetic, biological, and environmental factors make the investigation of the etiology of behavioral traits particularly complex. Most likely, progress in the determination of the etiology of many speech and language disorders will not be significant until models and investigations include all of these contributing factors. However, to determine the degree of contribution of a particular factor, that factor must be varied systematically while the other contributing factors are controlled. In some of the research models to be discussed in this book, the contribution of the genotypes is controlled and the environmental effects are varied, as in studies of monozygotes separated at birth, whereas in others the effect of the genotype is varied and the environmental effects are controlled, as in studies of adopted siblings with different biological parents.

DEFINITIONS OF THE PHENOTYPE

The simplest possible models assume a one-to-one correspondence between a single identifiable trait and a particular gene. Such a situation exists in the trisomy 21 form of Down's syndrome; the syndrome is distinctive, discontinuous from normal, is associated with physical characteristics as well as with cognitive abnormalities, and its expression is not markedly altered by psychosocial and environmental factors. In contrast, such a situation does not exist with any of the speech and language disorders we are considering in this volume. Children's language delay, stuttering, and dyslexia are all behavioral disorders, not associated with clear-cut physical abnormalities, and are syndromes where particular skills are at the extreme low end of the normal continuum.

Difficulties with the precise definition of these disorders present three major obstacles to those attempting to investigate a possible genetic basis for speech and language disorders. First, a criterion level of the behavior must be designated for determining when an individual exhibits the disorder (trait). Second, the presence or absence of behaviors associated with the major behavioral disorder must be defined objectively and criterion levels determined for each. Primary speech and language disorders are usually defined by "exclusion." That is, only when the speech and language disorders cannot be attributed to another defect which could have interfered with speech and/or language developments (e.g., deafness or mental retardation) can they be designated as primary. It is frequently the case that speech and language disorders co-occur with other behavioral disorders and that it is difficult to determine whether both are primary and independent disorders. Third, investigators must determine whether they will separate out various subtypes for independent study with the expectation that the various forms are independent traits or whether they will regard them as different expressions of the same trait. Thus, such a decision must be reached with respect to the disorders of stuttering and cluttering. Similarly, it is not known whether disorders such as developmental verbal dyspraxia and speech misarticulation represent different levels of severity of the same disorder or two separate disorders. In the developmentally language impaired, there is no one well accepted system for subtyping language impairment. Here the presence or absence of phonological disorders should perhaps be considered as signaling two different subtypes. Finally, types of dyslexia associated with impaired verbal functioning may need to be separated from those associated with visuospatial deficits.

Each decision regarding the definition of the phenotype to be studied must take into account two conflicting possiblities. If investigators have not separated two disorders that are indeed two different traits, then the different patterns of inheritance of these two will confound the results and interfere with their interpretation, possibly leading to an erroneous acceptance of the null hypothesis. On the other hand, if two disorders are really both expressions of a single trait, and differ as a result of environmental or other modifications of gene expression, they should be studied in combination. If only one is studied then the pattern of inheritance being examined will include only half the instances of the trait and hence may not become evident. Therefore, the decision as to whether two disorders are independent traits or different expressions of the same trait is a crucial one. In some areas, examination of epidemiological data is helpful prior to designing research on a group of disorders. However, the epidemiological data available on speech and language disorders is minimal (Leske, 1981), particularly regarding relative rates of co-occurrence of various speech and language disorders.

Given the state of the art, one approach in designing research in this area might be to define a disorder on the basis of objective and standardized tests with the aim of selecting the most discrete form that could possibly be a single trait. However, at the same time, the study should include procedures for identifying several different speech and language disorders. Thus, although subject ascertainment may be focused on one disorder, each of the other speech and language disorders occurring in the sample should be measured and included in the data base. The data can then be analyzed two ways to test whether these syndromes are separate traits or modified expressions of the same trait.

This approach assumes the availability of adequate measures for defining speech and language disorders. One of the major obstacles however for speech and language research in general, and genetic studies in particular, is the lack of such measures. Batteries of measures should include all behaviors contributing to linguistic performance and useful in identifying the areas of deficiency in speech and language development. Behaviors examined should include those which are found in the normal population and hence can be quantified both within the normal range and at the extreme ends of the continuum. In addition, those behaviors not found in the normal population (e.g., severe blocks noted in stuttering or excessive echolalia) should be assessed in order to identify subjects who represent a distinct and separate population. More generally, the criteria for determining when a patient is not normal and represents a different population need to be developed. In neurology, the Babinski reflex allows for the identification of pathology. An inventory of such signs for identifying speech and language pathologies would be of importance.

Because probands need to be identified at different ages, comparable measures across different ages need to be developed. As these are developmental disorders, their characteristics often change with development. For example, the behaviors that may be the most useful in identifying children with a particular syndrome at a given age level are those which are developing the most rapidly at that age in the normal population. Therefore, tests at each age level must allow for the assessment of behaviors most useful for the identification of a disorder at that age. In addition, tests must be standardized in reference to the normal population so that the degree of impairment relative to the normal population can be measured on the same metric across different ages. To illustrate, one should be able to determine whether a child is 2 standard performance deviations or more below normal performance in syntactic comprehension at ages 4–8. Further, family members of proband must also be measured on the same language behaviors as the proband to determine whether they exhibit the same pattern of performance. Thus normative data for the full age range are needed. The greatest gap at the present time is between the ages of 10 and 18 years, as few language tests with age-based norms exist in this range. Once such batteries of comprehensive measures are available, investigators will be able to search for the same phenotype in families by testing each family member. Also, the variabilities of expression of a particular phenotype could be assessed to determine how affected individuals differ and how the expression of the trait is related to factors that may be modifying expression.

In addition to problems of definition and measurement, the speech and language field also suffers from problems in terminology. Neurology and psychiatry, two disciplines dealing with behavioral disorders, have also been wrestling to varying degrees of success with this problem. The *Diagnostic and Statistical Manual of Mental Disorders, Third Edition (DSM-3)* of the American Psychiatric Association (1980) provides reference definitions for the identification of psychiatric disorders. These definitions are qualitative, and do not employ standardized measures. Definitions along these lines are needed in speech and language disorders but they should be based on objective standardized test measures. Thus comparisons could be made among data sets. However, such a situation does not appear readily forthcoming, and in the interim it would be an improvement at least to have some standard definitions of terms. For example, it needs to be made clear whether delayed language development, childhood dysphasia, and acquired aphasia are separate disorders; how they differ; and which terms are in fact synonymous.

In the medical tradition, the definition of disorders, or syndromes, is based on symptoms and the presence of pathological signs. Thus a list of symptoms or signs is usually sufficient for the identification of a disorder. The description of most speech and language disorders, however, is not so much based on the presence of certain symptoms or signs that do not occur within the normal population, as it is on the degree of deviation from the normally expected levels of certain behaviors or skills. This psychological approach to defining a disorder must also be included. Classification systems should, therefore, include both information on abnormal signs and symptoms and also definitions regarding the levels of speech and language behaviors within the normal population and the various disorders.

The identification of a speech and language syndrome often requires the exclusion of other developmental disabilities. To determine whether other developmental disorders may have contributed to the disorder observed in a speech-and-language-impaired person, these other disorders must be identified in a speech-and-language-impaired child. Valid measurement of perceptual, cognitive, and emotional factors in the speech-and-language-impaired population is often confounded. Therefore, it would be better to define a syndrome based on its characteristics rather than on the exclusion of other factors. This issue becomes particularly relevant when the definition of a characteristic trait is necessary for studies of speech and language disorders. Greater care should be taken, for example, in describing the characteristics of various reading disorders. This does not mean, however, that focus should be exclusively on the primary problem in defining a disorder. Clearly, those disorders secondary to other disorders (e.g., to mental retardation or psychiatric illness) should be excluded.

DELINEATION OF THE GENOTYPE

In attempting to define genotypes responsible for particular disorders, several different genetic research paradigms are available: adoption studies, twin studies, pedigree analysis, family studies, and genetic linkage studies. Each of these paradigms has a particular purpose; which should be used depends on the type of research question being asked and the available resources.

Pedigree analysis and genetic linkage analysis are most useful when genetic etiology of a disorder is already known and there is a need to identify the specific genetic mechanism. Twin and adoption studies are most useful for addressing questions regarding the relative contributions of genetic versus environmental and experimental factors. Twin studies, however, can be made more powerful when combined with family studies. Family studies can also be helpful in further defining the phenotype for study. By studying the affected and unaffected family members, it becomes possible to further define the specific symptoms and signs associated with the trait.

Speech and language functioning are highly affected by educational and socioeconomic factors. The rate and extent of development are particularly sensitive to environmental factors. However, it is not known to what extent environment or experience can alter speech and language disorders. Hence it is important to employ genetic paradigms that allow for the quantification of the effects of the environment on such disorders. For example, the study of adoptions of monozygotic twins reared in very different environments will demonstrate the effects of environment on these disorders (or skills). Here the genotype has been fixed and the environment varies. Further, if and when it is possible to identify a genetic marker for a trait, it becomes even more possible to examine the effects of environment and experience on that trait. Children with the marker are particularly interesting, as they can be followed through development, and environmental and experimental effects can be evaluated.

With our recent high divorce and remarriage rates, many half siblings and nonsiblings are being reared in the same environment and a significant number of biological siblings are being reared in different environments. Designs where half sibs or non-sibs are being reared together and biological sibs are being reared apart will allow for testing the roles of biological and environmental components. However, a major difficulty with these designs is the childhood emotional stress induced by a divorce or the death of a parent.

It can also be informative to study speech and language development when the genetic abnormality is well known. This approach has been used most successfully with sex chromosome abnormalities. If specific speech and language impairments can be found in genetic disorders they should be studied. This is particularly important when the speech and language deficiency is out of line with other cognitive and motor skills.

To identify which genetic abnormality is responsible for a particular disorder, one should also examine a large population with the disorder to determine the relative frequencies of other disorders in that population as compared to the normal population. Other types of disorders that are more frequent than in the general population might suggest a particular genetic locus which can affect each of these functions and produce different degrees of penetrance in various individuals.

Finally, genetic linkage studies are a relatively new tool. This approach will become much more powerful in the very near future (see Kimberling, this volume). It will be most useful with relatively rare, high-density, and multigenerational pedigrees that have been well characterized diagnostically. Blood samples for large families where a particular deficit has occurred over many generations should be reposited. With the newer, more powerful linkage techniques, many more of these studies can be conducted on such groups.

ANIMAL MODELS FOR RESEARCH ON GENETIC ASPECTS OF SPEECH AND LANGUAGE DISORDERS

At first glance the possibility of animal models for research aimed at determining the genetic bases of speech and language disorders seems limited at best. Certainly, there are no animal models for stuttering, dyslexia, or delayed language disorders. However, certain behavioral skills and learning can be studied in animals, and if some of these are found to be lateralized in the brain then they might have relevance to speech and language. If selective breeding were found to enhance such skills, then animal models could prove important. Control of bird song (Nottebaum, 1970), the detection of calls in monkeys (Petersen, Beecher, Zoloth, Moody, & Stebbins, 1978), and temporal discrimination in monkeys (Dewson, 1979) are all lateralized skills that have the greatest relationship to communicative abilities in humans. Hemispheric asymmetries in the length of the sylvian fissure have been demonstrated in chimpanzees (Yeni-Komshian & Benson, 1976). These anatomical asymmetries seem similar to those found in man and may be related to the lateralization of language in man. However, the critical link would be whether selective breeding can produce strains of animals with greater anatomical asymmetries and/or increased levels of skill in those behaviors that are lateralized in animals.

The rationale for developing animal models for research would be if such models could be used to address questions that cannot be addressed in human genetic research. Some of the pertinent questions that come to mind are whether hemispheric anatomical asymmetries have greater similarities in individuals with the same genetic material and whether they differ more between unrelated animals than they do between siblings or their parents. And, in strains with greater degrees of laterality, are behavioral patterns similarly affected? Finally, the development of animal strains with abnormalities for degree or pattern of laterality could be used to address the mode of inheritance and the genetic locus for such abnormalities.

To summarize, although the possibility of developing an appropriate animal model seems both difficult and controversial, such a model has great potential for furthering our understanding of genetic factors in the inheritance of anatomical and physiological differences. In addition, animal models might address whether extreme deviations in developmental learning and communication could be genetically based.

ACKNOWLEDGMENTS

This chapter includes a summary of the thoughts, suggestions, and concerns expressed by the participants in the Conference on Genetic Aspects of Speech and Language Disorders. Each of the following persons contributed to the ideas contained in this chapter: Eric Caine, Barton Childs, John DeFries, Roswell Eldridge, Joan Finucci, Al Galaburda, Norman Geschwind, Kenneth Kidd, William Kimberling, Herbert Lubs, David Mellits, Charles Netley, David Pauls, Paul Satz, Rachel Stark and Frank Wood.

REFERENCES

American Psychiatric Association. *Quick Reference to the Diagnostic Criteria from Diagnostic and Statistical Manual of Mental Disorders* (3rd ed.) Washington, DC: American Psychiatric Association, 1980.

Andrews, G., & Harris, M. *The Syndrome of Stuttering.* Lavenham, Suffolk: Lavenham Press, 1964.

Annell, A–L., Gustavson, K–H., & Tenstam, J. Symptomatology in schoolboys with positive sex chromatin (The Klinefelter Syndrome). *Acta Psychiatrica Scandinavica,* 1970, *46*, 71–80.

Arnold, G. E. The genetic background of developmental language disorders. *Folia Phoniatrica,* 1961, *13:* 246–254.

August, G. J., Stewart, M. A., & Tsai, L. The incidence of cognitive disabilities in the siblings of autistic children. *British Journal of Psychiatry,* 1981, *138*, 416–422.

Bartak, L., Rutter, M., & Cox, A. A comparative study of infantile autism and specific developmental receptive language disorder: I. The children. *British Journal of Psychiatry,* 1975, *126*, 127–145.

Bloodstein, O. Stuttering in families of adopted stutterers. *Journal of Speech and Hearing Disorders,* 1961, *26*, 395–396.

Bradford, D. Cluttering. *Folia Phoniatrica.* 1970, *22*, 272–279.

Brutten, E. J., & Shoemaker D. J. *The Modification of Stuttering.* Englewood Cliffs, N.J.: Prentice Hall, 1967.

Chakravartti, R., Roy, A. K., Rao, K. U. M., & Chakravartti, M. R. Hereditary factors in stammering. *Journal de Genetique Humaine,* 1979, *27,* 319–328.

Childs, B., & Finucci, J. M. The genetics of learning disabilities. *Human Genetics: Possibilities and Realities,* 1979, *66,* 359–376.

Cole, M. Specific educational disability involving spelling. *Neurology,* 1964, *14,* 968–970.

Decker, S. N., & DeFries, J. C. Cognitive abilities in families with reading disabled children. *Journal of Learning Disabilities,* 1980, *13,* 517–522.

Decker, S. N., & Defries, J. C. Cognitive ability profiles in families of reading disabled children. *Developmental Medicine and Child Neurology,* 1981, *23,* 217–227.

DeFries, J. C., Singer, S. M., Foch, T. T., & Lewitter, F. I. Familial nature of reading disability. *British Journal of Psychiatry,* 1978, *132,* 361–367.

Dewson, J. H. Toward an animal model of auditory cognitive function. In (C. L. Ludlow & M. E. Doran–Quine, Eds.), *The Neurological Basis of Language Disorders in Children: Methods and Directions for Research.* Bethesda, Md.: NINCDS Monograph Series, U.S. Department of Health, Education and Welfare, 1979.

Ehrman, L., & Parsons, P. A. *The Genetics of Behavior.* Sunderland, Mass.: Sinauer Associates, 1976.

Foch, T. T., DeFries, J. C., McClearn, G. E., & Singer, S. M. Familial patterns of impairment in reading disability. *Journal of Educational Psychology,* 1977, *69,* 316–329.

Folstein, S., & Rutter, M. Infantile autism: A genetic study of 21 twin pairs. *Journal of Child Psychology and Psychiatry and Allied Disciplines,* 1977, *18,* 297–321.

Freeman, F. J. Phonation in stuttering: A review of current research. *Journal of Fluency Disorders,* 1979, *4,* 78–89.

Funderburk, S. J., & Ferjo, N. Clinical observations in Klinefelter (47 XXY) Syndrome. *Journal of Mental Deficiency Research,* 1978, *22,* 207–212.

Garvey, M., & Mutton, D. E. Sex chromosome aberrations and speech development. *Archives of Disease in Childhood,* 1973, *48,* 937–941.

Gladstein, K. L., Seider, R. A., & Kidd, K. K. Analysis of the sibship patterns of stutterers. *Journal of Speech and Hearing Research,* 1981, *24,* 460–462.

Goldman, P. S. Development and plasticity of frontal association cortex in the infrahuman primate. In (C. L. Ludlow & M. E. Doran–Quine, Eds.), *The Neurological Bases of Language Disorders in Children: Methods and Directions for Research.* Bethesda, Md.: NINCDS Monograph Series, U.S. Department of Health, Education and Welfare, 1979.

Haka-Ikse, K., Stewart, D. A., & Cripps M. H. Early development of children with sex chromosome aberrations. *Pediatrics,* 1978, *62,* 761–766.

Hallgren, B. Specific dyslexia: A clinical and genetic study. *Acta Psychiatrica et Neurological,* 1950, Supplementum 65, 1–287.

Hier, D. B., Atkins, L., & Perlo, V. P. Learning disorders and sex chromosome aberrations. *Journal of Mental Deficiency Research,* 1980, *24,* 17–26.

Howard-Peebles, P. N., Stoddard, G. R., & Mims, M. G. Familial X-linked mental retardation, verbal disability and marker X chromosomes. *American Journal of Human Genetics,* 1979, *31,* 214–222.

Howie, P. M. Concordance for stuttering in monozygotic and dizygotic twin pairs. *Journal of Speech and Hearing Research,* 1981, *24,* 317–321. (a)

Howie, P. M. Intrapair similarity in frequency of disfluency in monozygotic and dizygotic twin pairs containing stutterers. *Behavior Genetics,* 1981, *11,* 227–238. (b)

Johnson, W. The Indians have no word for it. I. Stuttering in children. *Quarterly Journal of Speech,* 1944, *30,* 330–337.

Kaplan, A. R. *Human Behavior Genetics.* Springfield Ill.: Charles C Thomas, 1976.

Kidd, K. K., Heimbuch, R. C., & Records, M. A. Vertical transmission of susceptibility to stuttering with sex modified expression. *Proceedings of the National Academy of Sciences,* 1981, *78,* 1–658.

Kidd, K., Reich, T., & Kessler, S. A genetic analysis of stuttering suggesting single major focus. *Genetics,* 1973, *72:* s137.

Kimberling, W. J., & Brookhouser P. E. Biochemical and cytogenetic techniques for the study of communication disorders. *Laryngoscope,* 1981, *91,* 238–249.

LaBenz, P. J., & LaBenz, E. S. (Eds.). *Early Correlates of Speech, Language, and Hearing.* Littleton, Mass.: PSG Publishing Co., 1980.

Lenneberg, E. H. A biological perspective of language. In (E. H. Lenneberg, Ed.), *New Directions in the Study of Language.* Cambridge: MIT Press, 1964.

Leske, M. C. Prevalence estimates of communicative disorders in the US: Speech disorders. *ASHA.* 1981, *23,* 217–225.

Lewitter, F. I., DeFries, J. C., & Elston, R. C. Genetic models of reading disability. *Behavior Genetics,* 1980, *10,* 9–30.

Lockman, L. A., Swaiman, K. F., Drage, J. S., Nelson, K. B., Marsden H. M. *Workshop on the Neurobiological Basis of Autism.* NINCDS Monograph No. 23. Bethesda, Md.: U.S. Department of Health Education and Welfare, 1979.

Luchsinger, R. Inheritance of speech defects. *Folia Phoniatrica,* 1970, *22,* 216–230.

Mattejat, F., Niebergall, G., & Nestler, V. [Speech disorders in children of aphasic fathers: A developmental psycholinguistic case study.] *Praxis der Kinderpsychologie und Kinderspychiatrie.* 1980, *29,* 83–89.   (In German.)

McGlannan, K. K., Familial characteristics of genetic dyslexia: Preliminary report from a pilot study. *Journal of Learning Disabilities,* 1968, *1,* 185–191.

McLaughlin, J. F., & Kriegsman, E. Developmental dyspraxia in a family with X-linked mental retardation (Renpenning Syndrome). *Developmental Medicine and Child Neurology,* 1980, *22,* 84–92.

Mussafia, M. The role of inheritance in language and speech problems. *Folia Phoniatrica,* 1964, *16,* 228–238.

Mutton, D. E., & Lea, J. Chromosome studies of children with specific speech and language delay. *Developmental Medicine and Child Neurology,* 1980, *22,* 588–594.

Nielsen, J., & Sillesen, I. Follow-up till age 2–4 of unselected children with sex chromosome abnormalities. *Human Genetics,* 1976, *33,* 241–257.

Neilsen, J., Sorensen, A. M., & Sorensen, K. Mental development of unselected children with sex chromosome abnormalities. *Human Genetics,* 1981, *59,* 324–332.

Nottebaum, F. Ontogeny of bird song. *Science,* 1970, *167,* 950–956.

Omenn, G. S., and Weber, B. A. Dyslexia: Search for phenotypic and genetic heterogenity. *American Journal of Medical Genetics,* 1978, *1,* 333–342.

Pauls, D. L., & Kidd, K. K., Genetic strategies for the analysis of childhood behavioral traits. *Schizophrenia Bulletin,* 1982, *8,* 253–266.

Pennington, B., Puck, M., & Robinson, A. Language and cognitive development on 47XXX females followed since birth. *Behavior Genetics,* 1980, *10,* 31–41.

Petersen, M. R., Beecher, M. D., Zoloth, S. R., Moody, D. B., & Stebbins, W. C. Neural lateralization of species-specific vocalizations by Japanese macaques (*Macaca fuscata*). *Science, 202,* 324–326.

Porfert, A. R., & Rosenfield, D. B. Prevalence of stuttering. *Journal of Neurology, Neurosurgery, and Psychiatry,* 1978, *41,* 954–956.

Puck, M., Tennes, K., Frankenburg, W., Bryant, K., & Robinson, A. Early childhood development of four boys with 47 XXY karyotype. *Clinical Genetics,* 1975, *7,* 8–20.

Ratcliffe, S. G. Speech and learning disorders in children with sex chromosome abnormalities. *Developmental Medicine and Child Neurology,* 1982, *24,* 80–84.

Ross, A. D., & Pelham, W. E. Child psychopathology. *Annual Review of Psychology,* 1981, *32,* 243–278.

Sheehan, J. G., & Costley, M. S. A reexamination of the role of heredity in stuttering. *Journal of Speech and Hearing Disorders,* 1977, *42,* 47–59.

Siegel-Sadewitz, V. & Shprintzen, R. J. The relationship of communication disorders to syndrome identification. *Journal of Speech and Hearing Disorders,* 1982, *47,* 338–354.

Silver, L. B. Familial patterns in children with neurologically based learning disabilities. *Journal of Learning Disabilities,* 1971, *4,* 349–358.

Singer, S. M., Stewart, M. A., & Pulaski, L. Minimal brain dyfunction: Differences in cognitive organization in two groups of index cases and their relatives. *Journal of Learning Disabilities,* 1981, *14,* 470–473.

Spence, M. A. Genetic studies. In (E. R. Ritvo, Ed.), *Autism: Diagnosis, Current Research and Management.* New York: Spectrum, 1976.

Tennes, K., Puck, M., Bryant, K., Frankenburg, W., & Robinson, A. A developmental study of girls with trisomy X. *American Journal of Human Genetics,* 1975, *27:* 71–80.

Tuncbilek, E., Kurultay, N., & Belgin, E. Are sex chromosome abnormalities a factor in speech delay? *Archives of Disease in Childhood,* 1978, *53,* 831.

Valentine, G. H., McClelland, M. A., & Sergovich, F. R. The growth and development of four XYY infants. *Pediatrics.* 1971, *48*(4): 583–594.

Weiss, D. A. *Cluttering.* Englewood Cliffs, N.J.: Prentice Hall, 1964.

Yeni-Komshian, G. H., & Benson, D. A. Anatomical study of cerebral asymmetry in the temporal lobe of humans, chimpanzees, and Rhesus monkeys. *Science.* 1976, *192,* 387–389.

Zahalkova, M., Vrzal, V., & Kloboukova, E. Genetical investigations in dyslexia. *Journal of Medical Genetics,* 1972, *9,* 48–52.

Zaleski, T. [Familial appearance of delayed development of speech]. *Otolaryngologia Polska,* 1966, *20,* 367–371. (In Polish.)

Zimmerman, G. Stuttering: a disorder of movement. *Journal of Speech and Hearing Research* 1980, *23,* 122–136.

2

Genetics: Fate, Chance, and Environmental Control[1]

NORMAN GESCHWIND

Perhaps to many of the readers of this volume, some of the points I will make in this chapter will appear exceedingly trivial. Yet, the quality of many recent public discussions participated in even by distinguished biological scientists makes one realize that many of the elementary facts of genetics are not as well known as they should be. The extreme form of naiveté expressed by those who really do not know genetics is the view that one can assign traits either to totally determined genetic mechanisms or to effects of the environment. In addition, it is this naive view of genetics which leads many people to support extremely primitive notions of eugenics, for example, the notion that the only way to control a serious disorder is by eliminating those who carry the unfavorable gene. Another major form of naiveté concerning genetics is the view that every trait can be characterized as favorable, unfavorable, or neutral. Yet, as we shall see, there will be many instances in which a gene may be the bearer of alterations that may be *simultaneously* favorable and unfavorable, or that are favorable under some circumstances and unfavorable under others. It is, of course, also usually thought that if a particular gene leads to effects that are judged to be unfavorable, then surely it would be beneficial to eliminate it by some means. There may, however, be circumstances in which the advantage gained by the abolition of a gene may lead to favorable circumstances for a small group but to unfavorable ones for a much larger group. Although I have no pretensions at all to being a geneticist, I shall in this chapter highlight these

[1]Supported in part by the Orton Research Fund and the Essel Foundation Fund, and by grants from the National Science Foundation (BNS77-05674) and the National Institutes of Health (NS14018; NINCDS-06209).

21

and many other points which are perhaps not covered by other contributors to this volume who deal with more specific and substantive areas of genetics.

It may well be useful to begin this discussion with one of the favorite stories of Medawar, one of the giants of modern immunological investigation. In essence, Medawar asked his audience what they would think about a human patient who turned out to lack completely an enzyme that was absolutely necessary for the synthesis of a substance essential to normal bodily function and indeed to survival. Let us assume that a substance is discovered that will correct the adverse effects of this metabolic abnormality in such an individual. Two questions arise. In the first place, should one treat such an individual, or might it not be better for humanity in the long run to let him die of his disability? In the second place, if one decided that such a person should be kept alive, would it be reasonable to advise him not to have offspring, or indeed to prevent him from doing so by forceful measures? Most educated people believe that such a person should be given the appropriate therapy, but many would be in favor of attempting to convince him not to reproduce.

Yet, as Medawar pointed out, the condition he had in mind was the lack of the enzymatic systems necessary for the synthesis of vitamin C. This is, of course, a condition that is probably universal among humans (although it has occasionally been suggested that certain groups which are primarily car- nivorous might be exceptions). As it is obvious that one would not suggest that the entire human race abandon reproducing itself because of this genetic deficit, one must consider the implications of this example. In the first place, should one really deal differently with deficiencies that are not universal, but present in only a few people? Furthermore, one must realize that certain conditions of this kind might have compensatory advantages for those who are the bearers of the responsible genes, the elimination of which might thus confer no net benefit. There is another important implication of Medawar's example. It illustrates clearly the error of the belief that a genetic deficit condemns an individual to inevitable disability. Indeed, most of us enjoy the process by which we cure our own vitamin C deficiency and a large proportion of the population of California, Florida, and the Mediterranean area benefit from the existence of this genetic disorder.

This particular instance must also make us look carefully at the techniques for determining the respective contributions of genetics and environment to certain diseases. If citrus fruits were not generally available one might argue that that scurvy was an inherited disease. Yet, with universal use of vitamin C supplements one might not be aware that such a genetic disorder existed. It is also clear that many genetic disorders might be perfectly mimicked by environmental circumstances. Thus, consider an enzyme that is absolutely necessary for the manufacture from certain precursors of a substance essential for life. The disease that is caused by the lack of the final product would be observed in those who lack the enzyme. On the other hand, even those who have the enzyme will develop exactly the same disorder when the diet does not contain the necessary precursors on which the enzyme acts. Thus the presence or absence of a specific gene may be neither a necessary nor a sufficient condition for the occurrence of this disease.

Let me consider two further illuminating examples. Erway, Hurley, and Fraser (1966) studied mice with a dominantly inherited genetic disorder which led to failure of development of certain portions of the inner ear. They found, curiously, that this disorder could be produced in *all* the mice of this particular strain (including those who were *not* carriers of the gene) if the mother during pregnancy was placed on a *low* manganese diet, but that it did not appear in the offspring of noncarriers when the mother was on a "normal" manganese intake during pregnancy. A mouse who receives the gene from one or both parents will suffer from this disorder, even if the mother is on a *normal* manganese intake during the course of pregnancy. These authors then went on to show that in this case, the defect could be totally prevented in the offspring by placing the mother on a *high* manganese diet during pregnancy. Yet this maneuver did not abolish the genetic abnormality, as the expected proportion of the offspring of this pregnancy could be shown to carry the gene if they mated and the mother was placed on a *normal* manganese diet during pregnancy. If one were unaware of the effects of varying intake of manganese during pregnancy, the existence of generations in which the disease was not manifest might lead to failure to realize that the disorder was genetic, or to the conclusion that the inheritance was not dominant (since the mating of normal parents might give rise to affected offspring). Alternatively one might describe this condition correctly but purely descriptively as a dominant disorder with low or variable penetrance.

For the second example, let us consider a population a large percentage of whom suffered from a particular disease. One wishes to determine whether the disease is genetically or environmentally determined. One might employ the technique used by Kety and his co-workers in the study of schizophrenia; that is, one might determine the concordance in monozygotic and dizygotic twins. Assume that one finds a much higher concordance in monozygotic twins. One could go even further by means of the cross-fostering technique used by Kety and his co-workers in Denmark. Thus, one might find that the children of parents suffering from the disease still developed the disease in high frequency when they were adopted by foster parents not suffering from the disease, whereas children of parents who did not have the disease had a low incidence even when adopted by foster parents suffering from the disease. The conclusion that would generally be drawn is that the disease was predominantly genetically, rather than environmentally, caused. Suppose, however, that this hypothetical experiment were carried out in parts of Africa in which a large proportion of the population suffer from malaria. Carriers of the sickle cell trait will have malaria much less frequently than noncarriers. The children of carriers even when adopted by parents who themselves suffered from malaria, will tend to have a low frequency of the disorder, whereas the children of parents who had malaria will be more likely to contract the disease when adopted by parents free of the disease.

An even more striking example is found in the work of Miller et al. (1975). They pointed out that West Africans lack the Duffy blood group. Those who are Duffy negative have absolute resistance to vivax malaria, one of the four forms of this disorder. An adoption study would lead to dramatic results in areas in which this form of malaria was common and a significant proportion of the population were Duffy negative. These examples show that even dramatic "genetic" effects in an adoption study cannot rule out significant environmental pathogenesis of the disorder studied. One would not argue that malaria was inherited, since in the absence of a particular environmental pathogen, that is the malaria parasite, the disease does not occur. An adoption study can show only that genetics plays a role in pathogenesis. It cannot, however, distinguish between the circumstance in which an environmental pathogen is essential and what is inherited is susceptibility or resistance and the circumstance in which the disease might appear in those with appropriate inheritance regardless of environmental circumstances.

Even a structural abnormality of intrauterine origin may be absolutely dependent on an environmental factor, as in the experiments on the mice with "inherited" defects of portions of the inner ear. Another striking example appears in a paper by Millicovsky and Johnston (1981) who studied the A/J mouse. If an A/J mouse is given phenytoin at a certain time in pregnancy, nearly 100% of the offspring suffer from cleft lip and palate. In other strains of mice phenytoin does not have this effect, and therefore, A/J mice have an inherited susceptibility to this substance. If however the pregnant A/J mouse is placed in an atmosphere of *high* oxygen pressure after administration of phenytoin there is a sharp reduction of the incidence of cleft lip and palate. Conversely, a high percentage of offspring will have cleft lip and palate if an A/J mother who has *not* received phenytoin is exposed to *low* oxygen tension at the appropriate time.

Another often overlooked fact is that "genetic identity" does not necessarily determine identity or even similarity of the offspring. In many, perhaps most, cases, identical twins are discordant for various congenital anomalies as well as for later acquired diseases. Thus, there is discordance for juvenile diabetes in 50% of identical twin pairs (Rubinstein, Suciu-Foca, & Nicholson, 1977), and there is nearly 100% discordance for Parkinsonism. One should also be aware that many conditions that appear to be genetic are related to genetic constitution in a quite indirect way. Female rats but not male rats normally carry an enzyme that metabolizes steroids in a particular way. It is natural to think that such a circumstance is directly related to genes located on the sex chromosomes. Yet, the female given a single dose of androgen shortly after birth does not exhibit the enzyme in adult life and male rats castrated at birth, but not later in life, will have the enzyme, although in neither case is the genetic consitution altered. The critical feature is the presence or absence of circulating androgen at a certain time and not the sex chromosome genetic endowment itself.

One must also be careful to distinguish between *genetic* in the strict sense and *transmissible* (i.e., passed from mother to child and determined by factors other than those present in genes). Thus, cerebellar agenesis in cats is apparently the result of a virus which is transmitted from generation to generation. Beer and Billingham (1976) have pointed out that certain immune phenomena induced in a mother may be transmitted to succeeding generations. One of a pair of nonidentical twins may go through life with red blood cells that do not carry the genes that are present in his germ plasm or in any other cells of his body, but which were acquired in utero by transfusion from his sibling. Even the genes themselves are not immutable; like any other structural or chemical characteristic they can be deleted or changed by many external stimuli.

I have presented the preceding matters at length in order to make clear why I believe that it is important to look at the genetic causes of speech and language disorders. There is often strong resistance to the discussion of the role of genetic factors in many disorders, but in particular in those disorders that relate to behavior. Many feel that discussions of genetics are likely to lead to therapeutic nihilism, because of the common belief that if a condition is genetic it is neither correctable nor preventable, except by limitation of reproduction by carriers of the adverse genes. Furthermore, many will argue that even if there is a genetic component, it should be disregarded and stress should be placed on more practical and useful measures to overcome the inherited difficulties. My belief is, however, that these views are not "liberal," but rather misguided, and that the common existence of such views has served to inhibit research on genetic factors in many behavioral conditions. The reasons for studying genetics become obvious as soon as one realizes that genetics are not fate. Let me try to make this clear in the most elementary way. Discussions about genes on the part of most people—and, indeed, sometimes even on the part of sophisticated genetic researchers—embody what might be called the "strong" position. Thus, Stent (1981, p. 164) quotes the following statements from other authors: "[Genes] contain the information for the circuit diagram": "Genes blatantly specify the assembly of the nervous system . . . . Our 'only' questions, then, revolve around trying to find out *how* specific genes control neurobiological phenomena"; "Genes build nerve cells and specify the neural circuits which underlie behavior."

According to the "strong" position the action of the gene is rigidly programmed and only when a mutation occurs does that action alter. However, as the following brief consideration of some very basic principles should make clear, the strong position is untenable. The position I will take is not the result of a "liberal" attitude nor of a desire to achieve an ecumenical rapproachement between the nature and the nurture protagonists. My assertion is that there is no possible way to believe in the "strong" view unless one rejects the most elementary knowledge of chemistry.

Let us therefore specify what we mean by genetic endowment. Genes are chemical substances which happen to be transmitted from parents to offspring. They act in the same manner as other chemicals, that is, they participate in chemical reactions. In particular, the current view is that they play a large role in controlling the production of enzymes which in turn are involved in the production of particular substances.

A brief consideration will show that no gene can work independently of the environment. The rate of *any* chemical reaction without exception is a function of concentrations of reacting substances; presence or absence of catalysts (which are really only another form of reactant); pH; pressure; temperature; osmotic strength; rate of removal of the products, either by further chemical reactions or by transport out of the locus of the reaction; light; and the presence of other substances which may speed up, slow down, or alter the direction of the reaction. This list is probably incomplete, but it illustrates the point that the "environment" cannot be neglected.

Furthermore, the products of the reactions that are favored under certain conditions may be toxic. Yet this toxicity is itself chemical and can be altered by chemicals either produced by other bodily reactions or introduced from the outside.

In view of the potential modification of chemical reactions by so many environmental influences, it is surprising that genes are as reliable as they are. Any chemical engineer knows how difficult it is to ensure a consistent product from a series of chemical reactions.

It might be argued, however, that although the presence of a gene or genes does not guarantee that some particular series of chemical events will take place, nonetheless the *absence* of a gene must represent an immutable limitation on freedom. Yet even this is not always the case. Thus the lack of the genes that control the production of vitamin C is readily corrected by the external administration of the product of the missing reaction. In other instances the apparent absence of a gene is, in fact, illusory. In the rare disease hereditary angioneurotic edema there is normally a deficit of a particular substance called C1 esterase inhibitor. But treatment with danazol leads to normal levels of this substance. In other words, the patient does possess the gene and the cause of the disease is not absence of the gene but repression of its expression. There are several other examples of similar disorders.

One must admit, however, the possibility that in the absence of a gene necessary for the production of some enzyme that acts early in some metabolic cycle many subsequent biochemical steps may fail and may lead to the production of multiple anomalies. But even this does not constitute immutable fate as techniques are now being developed for the introduction of even large proteins into the nervous system. The effects of many genes may thus be totally counteracted by control of environmental circumstances or, alternatively, the deficiencies to which they lead can be corrected in many ways. In other words, the purpose of studying the genetics of speech and language disorders is to increase our capacity for preventing and treating these disorders.

It should be clear that what I have said is not a criticism of genetics as a science, but rather a strong expression of praise for it. The attributes of any organism are a result of wide variety of factors among which must be included the particular pieces of chemical machinery called genes which are passed on in the parental chromosomes. A knowledge of the full mechanism by which a trait is determined should eventually enable us to select parents who are likely to have affected children and to devise methods for prevention and cure of disabilities from which their offspring are likely to suffer. On the other hand, we must look at the possible advantages to the general population of the genetic endowments which may, in certain circumstances, have disadvantageous expression so as to avoid losing more than we gain by prevention or treatment of the unfavorable effects.

We must raise our level of sophistication about what is transmitted from the parent whether by genes or by any of the other mechanisms mentioned. Thus, Folstein and Rutter (1977) have shown that while identical twins are concordant for autism in 36% of cases (with 0% concordance for fraternal twins) the concordance rate rises to nearly 90% in identical twins when one considers not merely autism in the other member, but also other forms of developmental learning and behavioral disability such as dyslexia. Under these circumstances the concordance rate for the fraternal twins is only about 10%. It is necessary to be aware that there may be many different manifestations of the same genetic background.

I have pointed out that one must not assume without further investigation that certain genetic traits are purely unfavorable. Many such traits can confer significant advantages under different environmental conditions. This is especially true for recessive genes that confer an advantage on the heterozygote. Sickle cell trait, with its protection against malaria, and sickle cell anemia, with its devastating effects, are obvious examples. Yet, the advantage of a trait may totally vanish under other circumstances; for example, resistance to malaria is of little or no advantage in most of the advanced countries in the world.

Even the individual who is suffering from certain defects may simultaneously possess important advantages. In illiterate societies those people who in our society are dyslexic might well have had important advantages in terms of their frequent superior mathematical and spatial functions. We must ask whether the total prevention of dyslexia is necessarily desirable if it also leads to a sharp reduction in the frequency of certain other talents. Sufferers from certain disorders may have very important compensatory talents; the relatives of these patients who share much of the same genetic constitution often possess the high talents in the absence of the unfavorable effects. Thus, many dyslexics have highly important artistic, musical, mathematical, and atheltic talents which may well be closely linked to the very same circumstances which produced the dyslexia itself. Furthermore, the close relatives of dyslexics may be endowed with precisely the same talents in the absence of any significant learning disability. This is particularly likely to be true of the female relatives, so that one commonly sees the pattern in which many male relatives do suffer from learning disabilities, whereas the females either lack these entirely or have them in only mild degree while still possessing all of the compensatory abilities.

Patients suffering from manic–depressive illness often have records of significant accomplishment and they may continue to be extremely productive in periods of freedom from illness. Andreasen and Kanter (1974) found, in a fascinating study of talented authors, that their relatives have a high frequency of both affective illness and superior endowment. Heston (1966) found that the unimpaired siblings of schizophrenics tended to be more spontaneous and creative than controls. Karlson (1970) reported that the close relatives of psychotics have a significantly increased probability of being considered eminent. I am not suggesting that we will necessarily find ourselves in the difficult position of being unable to prevent the occurrence of any or all of these disabilities without sacrificing a disproportionate number of valuable talents. Rather, I am arguing that it is only by gaining detailed knowledge of the genetic mechanisms and of the environmental modifying influences, both in pre- and postnatal life, that we will be able to develop effective methods of prevention or amelioration of these disabilities, while retaining the favorable effects of the genes carried by these individuals.

Another major reason for the study of the genetics of speech and hearing disorders is that genetic study will potentially make available animal experimental models. In nearly all branches of medicine animal models have repeatedly proved essential in clarifying the mechanisms of abnormal conditions and providing new approaches to therapy. Yet, in the field of the more complex behavioral attributes of humans it has usually been believed that this type of approach was not available. How could one study language, psychosis, and artistic, mathematical, and musical talents in other species, in which the relevant abilities appear to be if not largely, completely, lacking? If rats or monkeys cannot learn to read how can we possibly study the pathogenesis of dyslexia in these species? A little reflection shows that there are potentially powerful methods for use of these nonhuman species despite apparently insuperable barriers.

Two methodologies are particularly promising. The first is the study of the structural foundations of communicative abilities in the nervous system. The second is the study of genetic mechanisms. The two methodologies are not unrelated, but I will stress here the importance of genetics. One of the major contributions of genetics has been to teach us again and again to distinguish carefully between the phenotype (i.e., the external manifestations) and the underlying mechanisms. As Stent (1981) has so brilliantly pointed out, one has to distinguish carefully between the final perceptible manifestations of the presence of genes and the underlying mechanisms. Thus, at first glance it appears that the Siamese cat frequently carried genes for crossed eyes. Yet closer inspection shows that the genes involved probably have no primary direct effect on the systems controlling the position of the eyes. The crossed eyes of the Siamese cat are probably the secondary result of the anomalous organization of the visual cortex. As Stent argues, it is unlikely that the genes involved primarily affect the visual cortex itself; the alterations in this structure are probably secondary to maldevelopment of the pigment epithelium of the retina. Even this mechanism is probably not primary since the abnormal development of the pigment epithelium is itself the result of an alteration in the formation of pigmented cells which also manifests itself in the albino coat coloring of this strain of cats. In other words, one might begin by studying the inheritance of crossed eyes in the albino animal, but a persistent search for underlying mechanisms eventually leads to a consideration of the effect of genes that control enzymes involved in the production of melanin.

In the same fashion, we must use the clues provided by genetics and structure to shift our discussion of the genetics of dyslexia, stuttering, autism, schizophrenia, manic–depressive illness, and other disabilities to a level at which we are considering the control of mechanisms that underlie the structure and chemistry of the nervous system. It is my belief that at this more basic level we are very likely to find that many of the mechanisms that lead to these behavioral disorders in humans are in fact at play in other species. In some instances, we may find that in these species similar fundamental mechanisms may lead to a series of traits which at the superficial external level appear to be totally different from those manifested in humans. Alternatively, we may find that despite the absence of spontaneous alterations of this type in other species, it may be possible to devise experimental methods that act on precisely the same basic mechanisms. If we can reach these goals, then the study of even very distant species may well provide us with investigative procedures which will clarify the mechanisms of these disorders in humans and perhaps lead to therapeutic techniques.

Let me now turn to another issue that overlaps very closely with much that I have already said. Like any other part of scientific investigation, the study of transmissible traits (I use this phrase specifically in order to indicate that one must consider not only mechanisms controlled directly by genes, but also other mechanisms such as I have already described) has many pitfalls. I have already pointed out that it is an error to assume that even complete knowledge of the complement of the genes carried by an organism will enable us to predict with full accuracy its structure or its behavior. Thus, as Stent has pointed out, even among leading figures in the world of genetics there have been major disagreements as to what information such complete knowledge would provide. Although certain investigators hold that the genetic endowment would completely specify the structure of the nervous system, many others have argued against this view. Stent reminds us that even in simple nervous systems which contain only a few hundred or a few thousand neurons there may be considerable varability in the number of neurons, their position, and their connections, depending on chance environmental events.

If chance events are important sources of variability in simple nervous systems, they must play an even greater role in higher organisms. Several examples have already been discussed on p. 24. Another illustrative case is that of the preoptic nucleus in the rat. This set of neurons appears to control the cyclic release of gonadotropins in females (which leads to the occurrence of a menstrual cycle) which is lacking or much less marked in males. This functional difference is related to sexual dimorphism, that is, the male and female preoptic nuclei differ in structure. One might have assumed that the structural differences were fully specified by variations in genetic endowment. Yet, if the newborn female rat receives a large single injection of testosterone, she will not have an estrus cycle and her preoptic nucleus will assume the typical male form. By contrast, if the newborn male rat is castrated, his preoptic nucleus will release gonadotropic hormones cyclically in adult life and will manifest the typical female morphology. Thus environmental events can markedly modify the final form of the nucleus. Another possible hypothesis is that the organism contains genes that can lead to either the typical female or the typical male pattern. The pattern selected will depend on chemical events which repress or release one or the other of these gene systems at some critical period. This does not, however, argue against the conclusion that the original gene endowment alone cannot determine the final form, but rather supports it.

Furthermore, at least in mammals, certain events occurring shortly before or shortly after birth, must favor variability of the final structural and chemical pattern of the brain. It is known that in many species there is a marked overproduction of cells in the fetal brain. Extensive cell death takes place in the late prenatal and early postnatal periods when neurons that fail to establish connections are lost. This mechanism of this type may explain why many genetic disorders manifest themselves in different ways. As King (1936) pointed out, hereditary agenesis of the corpus callosum is present in certain mice. Yet, within the same family one may find remarkable degrees of variation in the extent and precise form of this abnormality.

Misunderstanding results from the common expectation that it is easy to specify Mendelian patterns of inheritance simply by study of family lineages. Yet, as is well known to geneticists, deviations from classic Mendelian patterns are common. Cytoplasmic or extrachromosomal inheritance does not follow Mendelian patterns because only the mother transmits cytoplasmic genes. Even when traits depend on genes located on chromosomes, there may be apparently confusing patterns of transmission. It has been argued for many years that torsion dystonia, a disorder of Eastern European Jewish children, is inherited as a sex-linked recessive character. At least one group of investigators have now argued that the mode of inheritance is autosomal dominant.

How could such wide discrepancies of interpretation appear even among experts? There are several mechanisms which may lead to such problems in interpretation. As the work of Erway et al. (1966) shows, a dominantly inherited disorder may be completely absent in one generation, yet reappear in the offspring. The almost exclusive occurrence of certain disorders in males may be the result of sex-linked inheritance, but it may also occur when certain factors modify expression in females. If disorders are present at one period, but disappear later, a genetic analysis that does not take account of age may lead to mistaken conclusions. Bray and Wiser (1964) studied the inheritance of sylvian seizures. If EEG's were done on the parents of such patients one might conclude that the disorder was recessive, because the parents only infrequently showed any abnormality. The entire picture changes when it is realized that this abnormality frequently disappears in adolescence. Bray and his co-workers concluded that this particular trait was in fact inherited as an autosomal dominant.

Another problem arises when some individuals who inherit the genes for some disorder die in intrauterine life. In this case study of living patients with the abnormality may give a skewed genetic pattern. Another curious pattern is seen in Huntington's chorea. Childhood onset cases are usually transmitted by the father. A hypothesis entertained at one time was that when the mother was the affected parent a higher percentage of the fetuses die. It turns out however, that a quite different mechanism is at work. When the mother is affected the disease is likely to occur later in adult life. In myotonic dystropy one finds the reverse pattern in childhood onset cases (i.e., predominant transmission from the mother).

There are many other examples of such pitfalls. I have already alluded to the high rate of nonconcordance for diseases and traits among identical twins. On the other hand, it is often asserted that dizygotic twins are no more alike than any other two siblings. Yet, dizygotic twins are less likely to reject skin grafts from each other than are other pairs of siblings. Furthermore, as has been mentioned, a dizygotic twin may actually carry not only the kind of red cells determined by the genes that he received from his parents, but also the type of red cells carried by his twin. Furthermore, many issues regarding resemblances among twins and the mechanisms of twinning remain unclear. One would expect that in identical twin pairs, both members would be right-handed or both would be left-handed. Yet, pairs in which one member is right-handed and one member is left-handed are common—indeed, more common than pairs in which both are left-handed. This raises important questions about an issue that is relevant to the genetic and environmental factors controlling cerebral lateralization. Curiously enough, problems almost identical in form may exist among much lower species. Larrabee (1906) found in trout that the optic nerve coming from the right eye lies dorsal to the left in the majority of cases. This population asymmetry had no obvious genetic background, since trout parents in both of whom the right optic nerve was dorsal were no more likely to have offspring with this pattern than any other combination of parents. Even more perplexing were the findings in two-headed trout monsters. Larrabee assumed that the two heads should have precisely the same genetic pattern. The actual findings did not fit this assumption. Thus, in 33% of cases both heads had the right nerve dorsal, in 14% both left dorsal, and in 53% the pattern was discordant in the two heads. The distribution of the right or left dorsal positions in the two heads was, as the author did not realize, exactly the same distribution that would have occurred in random pairs of unrelated trout! Larrabee found these findings so perplexing that he concluded that the results were purely random, but it is difficult to accept such a conclusion. Seventy-five years later we are still perplexed by many of the same issues of inheritance of lateralization. Indeed, it has been argued by some investigators that the handedness in monozygotic twin pairs follows exactly the same distribution that would be found in pairs of unrelated individuals in the population chosen at random!

Finally, we must remember that, particularly in the field of behavior, it is easy to be trapped into assuming that anything that has a name and is apparently measurable can be studied genetically. The major objection to studies of the inheritance of IQ is not the question of culture-bound tests, but rather the fact that the very concept of inheritance of the overall IQ is probably incorrect. As IQ tests contain many subtests, and an individual's performance across subtests may vary greatly, it is likely that we are dealing with sets of independent abilities and that the overall score itself cannot be regarded in any useful way as a genetic trait. Consider the analogous problem of a test of overall athletic ability. It is not possible to create a metric that compares a 95-pound female gymnast and a 250-pound fullback. The notion of the inheritance of "general" intelligence is probably as faulty as that of the inheritance of some mysterious quality of "athletic ability."

Similarly, the mere existence of a method of measurement does not insure that the numbers obtained correspond to biological reality. Considerable effort has been expended on measuring the "heritability" of certain traits. Yet the preceding discussion shows that possibly every genetic trait is capable of complete suppression or complete expression depending on the environment. The heritability of a trait is thus not a fixed property of the trait but rather one that varies under different environmental conditions. That such a measure may have a limited usefulness as a kind of practical engineering measure cannot be denied, but too often it obscures clear thinking about basic mechanisms.

It is often equally misleading to attempt to prove that some disorder has a genetic contribution to its pathogenesis. Such a study can be useful but its limitations must be kept in mind. Can one name a disorder that has no genetic contribution? Consider fractures. If one were to consider—obviously only in thought!—an experiment in which people were dropped out of second-story windows would one not find that the distribution of fractures had an important genetic contribution? Would not identical twins be more likely to have a similar number and type of fractures than two unrelated individuals? What we really want to know is the detailed pathogenesis of any disorder which will include the inherited chemicals in the chromosomes and the full array of other influences.

Our purpose is to understand what leads to developmental disorders of speech and language. The great advantage of looking at genetics is to open wide a biological door that has behind it many unexpected facts that may throw light on the detailed mechanisms that we wish to understand.

REFERENCES

Andreasen, N., & Kanter, A. The creative writer: Psychiatric symptoms and family history. *Comprehensive Psychiat.* 1974, *15,* 123–131.

Beer, A. E., & Billingham, R. *The immunobiology of mammalian reproduction.* Englewood Cliffs, N.J.: Prentice-Hall, 1976.

Bray, P., & Wiser, W. C. Evidence for a genetic etiology of temporal-central abnormalities in focal epilepsy. *New England Journal of Medicine,* 1964, *271,* 926–933.

Erway, L., Hurley, L. S., & Fraser, A. Neurological defect: Manganese in phenocopy and prevention of a genetic abnormality of inner ear. *Science,* 1966, *152,* 1766–1768.

Folstein, S., & Rutter, M. Genetic influences on infantile autism. *Nature,* 1977, *265,* 726–278.

Heston, L. Psychiatric disorders in foster home reared children of schizophrenic mothers. *Brit. J. Psychiat.,* 1966, *112,* 819–825.

Karlsson, J. Genetic association of giftedness and creativity with schizophrenia. *Hereditas,* 1970, *66,* 177–182.

King. L. A. Hereditary defects of the corpus callosum in the mouse, *Mus musculus. Journal of Comparative Neurology,* 1936, *64,* 337–363.

Larrabee, A. P. The optic chiasma of teleosts: A study of inheritance. *Proc. Amer. Acad. Arts and Sciences,* 1906, *12,* 217–231.

Miller, L. H., Mason, S. J., Dvorak, J. A., McGinnis, M. H., & Rothman, I. K. Erythrocyte receptors for (*Plasmodium knowlesi*) malaria: Duffy blood group determinants. *Science,* 1975, *189,* 561–563.

Millicovsky, G., & Johnston, M. C. Maternal hyperoxia greatly reduces the incidence of phenytoin-induced cleft lip and palate in A/J mice. *Science,* 1981, *212,* 671–672.

Rubinstein, P. L., Suciu-Foca, N., & Nicholson, J. F. Genetics of juvenile diabetes mellitus. *New England Journal of Medicine,* 1977, *297,* 1036–1040.

Stent, G. S. Strength and weakness of the genetic approach to the development of the nervous system. *Annual Review of Neuroscience,* 1981, *4,* 163–194.

II

DEFINING THE PHENOTYPE

3

Behavioral Attributes of Speech and Language Disorders

RACHEL E. STARK
E. DAVID MELLITS
PAULA TALLAL

INTRODUCTION

If genetic studies of speech and language disorders in children are to be
carried out, it will be necessary to define these disorders behaviorally and to find
a means of identifying the children who present them or are at-risk for developing them. These tasks are not simple. There are a number of possible approaches to the identification of speech and language disorders in children, but
none are completely straightforward.

The simplest approach is to ask parents whether or not their children are
speech or language impaired. Most, although not all, children diagnosed as
language impaired are reported by their parents as having speech or language
problems. However, many children who are considered by parents or clinicians
to be speech or language impaired in early childhood overcome these problems and are not so identified in their later school years.

Another approach is to employ standard tests and measurements of speech
and language. Usually, a normal underlying distribution of abilities in speech and
language is assumed for the construction of these tests. Thus, speech and
language impairment has to be defined in terms of a cutoff score (e.g., two
standard deviations from a given mean score) or of a degree of deficit (e.g.,
"language age more than 1 year below chronological or mental age.") When
continuous measurements are employed in this manner, however, the definitions
of speech or language impairment may become somewhat arbitrary. Also, as
existing standardized tests are not entirely satisfactory and as scores on any

GENETIC ASPECTS OF
SPEECH AND LANGUAGE DISORDERS

standard test are subject to error, a child may fall into a low normal category at one time and into an impaired category at another.

A third approach would be to examine groups of children for whom a clinical judgment of severe and persisting speech or language impairment had been made and to derive a set of criteria capable of identifying such children reliably. In this case, the measures employed would be discrete rather than continuous, and the speech- and language-impaired children would be treated as falling into a clearly different and separate group from their peers. Such a group might be heterogeneous and difficult to characterize.

Finally, it would also be possible to examine the patterns of deficit in language-related abilities (e.g., perceptual and motor abilities) that are characteristic of language-impaired children. In this manner, variables might be identified that would serve to discriminate normal from language-impaired children. It is possible, however, that perceptual–motor deficits, although included in the complete range of phenotypic expression of a particular gene defect, are not necessarily accompanied by speech and/or language disorders. They might serve as markers for affected families rather than identifying characteristics of speech- or language-impaired children.

ACQUISITION OF LANGUAGE IN NORMAL AND SPEECH- AND LANGUAGE-DISORDERED CHILDREN

The effectiveness of these approaches to identification of speech- and language-impaired children may vary greatly with the age of the child. All may be more difficult to apply in the preschool years because of the extreme variability in rate of language acquisition among normal children in this age range. Thus, Morley (1965), in a study of approximately 1000 children in Newcastle, England, showed that children who were ultimately indistinguishable with respect to language and learning abilities acquired the production of words and phrases over a wide range of ages. The range for first-word acquisition in these normal children was 6–30 months; for phrases, the range was 10–44 months. These findings indicate that preschool children with normal potential for language may quite readily be misidentified as having speech and language problems, both by parental report and by standard speech and language measures. Because of the great variability in attainment of early language milestones, the numbers of children who could be so misidentified may be significant. In a recent study, for example, conventional testing methods resulted in estimates of significant speech and language delay in over 25% of all preschool children (Allen & Bliss, 1979). By first grade, the estimates of speech and language delay tend to be much lower, approximately 6% (Marge, 1972).

Rates of acquisition of different units of language (e.g., of phonemes, words, and multiword utterances) are represented in Figure 3.1 by means of an idealized function. For the purpose of this chapter the figure will be interpreted

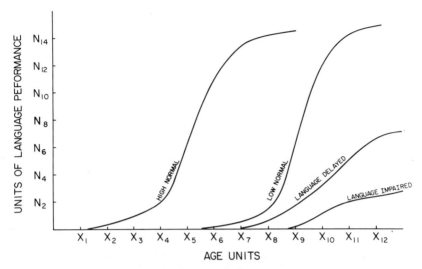

FIGURE 3.1. Idealized function representing the acquisition of units of language performance with age in normal, language-delayed, and language-impaired children.

as illustrating the acquisition of single words. On the left we see an idealized function for acquisition of single-word production in normally developing children. Initially, normal children acquire words slowly, some words being used for a short time only and then dropped. Subsequently, there is a marked spurt in vocabulary growth without loss of new items. Periods of less rapid growth may follow.

Real data of this kind are presented in Figures 3.2 and 3.3. Figure 3.2 (from Morley, 1965) shows average growth functions based upon percentages of normal children acquiring production of words, phrases, and intelligible speech at different ages. Figure 3.3 (from Brown, Cazden, & Bellugi, 1970) illustrates the growth of utterance length with age in three normal children. Clearly, this growth is not uniform within the individual child but is marked by temporary lapses as well as by spurts. The figure also illustrates the variability in acquisition of stages or milestones among individual normal children.

Returning to Figure 3.1, the next function represents word acquisition in a group of children who are eventually normal in all aspects of speech and language and in verbal learning, but who are markedly delayed in the earliest stages of language acquisition.

The third function in Figure 3.1 represents word acquisition in children who may be at the lower extreme of a normal distribution in this respect. Such children may be identified by their scores on standard tests of speech and language in relation to the scores of a population of children of the same age and socioeconomic status.

Real data of this kind, again from Morley (1965), are shown in Figure 3.4. The data are from a study of children with delayed development of articulation

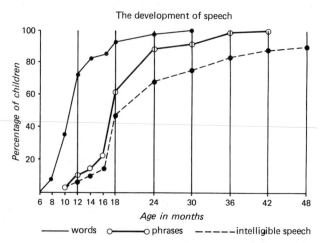

FIGURE 3.2. Percentage of normal children acquiring words, phrases, and intelligible speech from 6 to 48 months of age. (From M. Morley, *The development and disorders of speech in childhood*, London: Livingstone, 1965.)

of speech and represent the percentages of children from this group acquiring production of words, phrases, and intelligible speech at different ages.

Language-delayed children continue to acquire speech and language skills in their preadolescent years. Some may eventually be capable of academic success, particularly in science and mathematics. Others may reach a developmental plateau in verbal skills early in the school years and may go on to fail in academic subjects or to be labeled as "low achievers." Standard tests administered in early school years may not be good predictors of such outcomes, however. As in the case of cognitive abilities, the older the child, the greater the predictive value of standardized speech and language measures.

The last function in Figure 3.1, on the extreme right, represents the acquisition of single-word productions by language-impaired children. These children differ from language-delayed children. Their ability to produce many of the components of language and their speech intelligibility are severely depressed. They may show very slow rates of growth and early plateaus for language abilities in comprehension, in production, or in both. It might be concluded that a set of criteria for the identification of these children could be developed quite readily. As is suggested by the idealized functions in Figure 3.1, however, it may be difficult in the early preschool years to discriminate the three initially delayed groups from one another. In addition, although the judgment of language impairment may be an obvious one after the child reaches the age of 3–4 years, it may be quite difficult to develop criteria that would distinguish the language-impaired child from the child who has significant mental retardation or a pervasive developmental disorder. In addition, language-impaired children may form a more heterogeneous group than language-delayed children. They may show

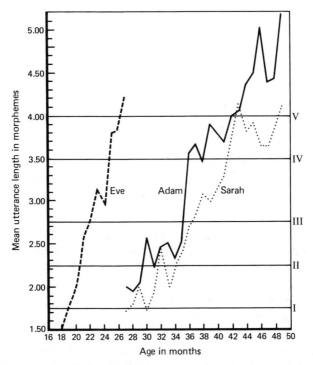

FIGURE 3.3. Growth in mean length of utterance with age in three normal children. (From Roger Brown, Courtney Cazden, & Ursula Bellugi, The child's grammar from I to III, in J. P. Hill (Ed.), *Minnesota symposium on child psychology*, 1969; reprinted in Roger Brown, *Psycholinguistics: Selected papers*, New York: Free Press, 1970.)

more uneven or deviant developmental profiles for language and cognitive abilities than the language-delayed group and may have severe difficulty in adapting to educational environments. They may come to be functionally retarded as a result.

Why is it that some children—including children who are later found to be normal—are markedly delayed in language acquisition? It has been suggested that young children may show a variety of cognitive styles and strategies in language acquisition. A number of investigators have identified subgroups among normal preschool children who employ "expressive," "imitative," or "referential/analytic" strategies in acquiring language (e.g., K. N. Nelson, 1973; Ingram, 1983; K. E. Nelson, 1981). It may be that in some cases the child's strategy is not compatible with the interactive style of the mother. The child may persist in employing an inappropriate strategy (from his mother's standpoint) for several months and as a result may show a temporary delay in language acquisition.

Alternatively, it has been proposed that young children may differ considerably with respect to the development of language-related skills. Differences in

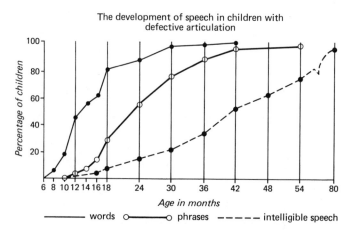

FIGURE 3.4. Percentage of children with defective articulation of speech, acquiring words, phrases, and intelligible speech from 6 to 80 months of age. (From M. Morley, *The development and disorders of speech in childhood,* London: Livingstone, 1965.)

the growth of speech discrimination, of short-term auditory memory, of motor sequencing and sequencing of the movements for speech, of motor coordination, of subtle cognitive or representational abilities, or of the ability to employ hierarchical ordering in perception or production of speech—any of these might contribute to delays in the comprehension or production of spoken language. Thus, the marked but quite temporary delay in language learning in the normal child may reflect delay in acquiring a particular skill or aspect of development. When the child attains a certain threshold level with respect to that skill, he may suddenly begin to understand the uses and nature of language more clearly. The skill that developed more slowly may become integrated with other, more rapidly developing, skills and there may then be an acceleration in language development.

According to this view, the child who is truly *language delayed* might develop some or all of the perceptual and motor abilities related to language at a much slower rate than children in either normal group. He, too, may develop language acquisition strategies that are not compatible with the interactive styles of his family members or his teachers. Unlike the normal child who is initially delayed but catches up with his peers, the language-delayed child, however, may fail to integrate certain basic aspects of language until much later in the school years. He may continue to develop language at a slower than normal rate, and may experience difficulty in learning in later school grades.

The child who is severely *language impaired* may present a greater number of deficits in perceptual and motor skills related to language, or a few deficits of this type that are more basic or are of exceptional severity. His deficits may also include difficulty in interacting with others, and may be based upon significant neurological impairment.

PERCEPTUAL AND MOTOR DEFICITS IN
SPEECH- AND LANGUAGE-DISORDERED CHILDREN

A study was designed to examine sensory, perceptual, and motor abilities in speech- and language-delayed and in normal school-aged children (Stark & Tallal, 1980). The initial identification of speech- and language-delayed children was an important aspect of the study. The purpose of the study was specifically to determine if there were perceptual and motor correlates of language delay or impairment that might suggest etiological factors. It was hoped that the study might also suggest new intervention strategies.

The children were 5–8½ years in age; they were selected in such a manner as to yield a specifically language-delayed group, a speech-articulation-delayed group (without significant language delay), and a normal control group. The children in the two delayed groups had already been identified by teachers and clinicians as having difficulty with speech and language and they were receiving treatment for their speech and/or language deficits. None of the children in the study were hearing impaired or presented a history of hearing impairment. None were significantly disordered in their behavioral or emotional development and none were neurologically impaired. From among the children initially selected, a further selection was made by means of standardized tests, as described in Stark and Tallal (1981). All of the children selected were of normal nonverbal intelligence (performance IQ greater than 85). The language-delayed children were required to be functioning, in receptive and expressive language, below the level that would be expected on the basis of their performance mental age (Wechsler, 1963, 1974). The speech-delayed children had significant problems with articulation of speech, but had receptive and expressive language abilities within the normal range.

The process of selection was impeded by the fact that an accepted battery of language tests, suitable for the identification of language impaired children, does not yet exist. A language scale, similar to the WISC-R or WPPSI scales for measurement of intelligence, would be useful for this purpose. In the absence of such a scale, it was necessary to use existing standardized tests and to derive weighted scores indicating level of receptive and of expressive language (Stark, Tallal, & Mellits, 1982). On the basis of these indices a group of children were identified that were delayed by more than 1 year in linguistic abilities. It should be noted that some, although not all, of these children also had speech articulation impairment as well. The children in the speech-delayed group were functioning at least 1 year below age level in speech articulation ability but were not delayed in receptive or expressive language. It is probable that some of the language-delayed children selected, those who were most severely impaired, would have fallen into our hypothetical language-impaired group in Figure 3.1. Others, those who were less severely impaired, might best be described as language delayed. For the purposes of the present account, however, this entire group of children will be referred to as language delayed.

First, it may be of interest to ask, could these children have been selected on the basis of parents' reports of speech and language disorder alone? It appears that they could not. At least 6 of the language-delayed children and 20 of the speech-delayed children were reported to have shown normal development of language milestones throughout the preschool years. Of the 6 language-delayed children, 2 came from homes of lower socioeconomic status, where the parents may have been accepting of their children's delayed speech and language. It is also possible that cultural biases in existing speech and language tests contributed to their poor performance on these tests; however, they were considered by their teachers to be functioning significantly below their classmates in language abilities. The remaining 4 language-delayed children who had been reported as having language milestones in the normal range were considered by their parents to be inept in social interaction rather than linguistically impaired. In addition, one of the children in the normal group was reported as delayed in language in the preschool years.

Could the speech- and language-delayed children have been selected on the basis of the judgments of teachers and clinicians alone? For the purposes of the study to be described, such judgments were more successful in identifying speech-delayed than language-delayed children. It was found, for example, that some children who had been identified as language delayed were mildly to moderately retarded, with verbal IQ and performance IQ both being depressed; others were mildly hearing impaired or had a history of middle ear disease; one was neurologically impaired; and a few children no longer manifested significant delay in language. Thus, the use of standardized tests, including tests of intelligence and of hearing, and neurological evaluation, proved to be important in identifying children for this study, above and beyond the reports of parents, teachers, and clinicians. It may be, however, that the definition of speech and of language disorder used in this study was more restricted than would be necessary for genetic studies.

It might also be asked, then, how accurate were standardized speech and language measures in this study in identifying children with persisting language impairment? It must be remembered that such measures were used in conjunction with the clinical judgment of teachers and speech and language pathologists. In a follow-up study of children identified in this manner it was found that almost all had residual problems in expressive language, especially in naming, and most were significantly impaired in reading. However, it was also found that some of the children were no longer significantly delayed in receptive language functioning. Specifically, those children who were youngest (5 to 7 years) at the time of initial contact formed a heterogeneous group with respect to residual problems, some remaining significantly impaired and others showing improvement. In contrast, the children who were oldest (8–8½) years at the time of initial contact remained significantly language impaired. They were still significantly below normal in expressive and receptive language functioning and in reading at the time of follow-up.

The children in the original study were selected so that, by proportional sampling, the three groups—normal, speech delayed, and language delayed—were very similar in age, performance IQ, race, and socioeconomic status. The children in all three subject groups were given an extensive battery of experimental perceptual and motor tests. These included tests of auditory identification, sequencing, rapid rate sequencing, and serial memory; visual and cross-modal identification, sequencing, rapid rate sequencing, and serial memory; and oral stereognosis. A neurodevelopmental battery and a speech motor battery were also administered. Although children found by medical history or classical neurological examination to be neurologically impaired were excluded from the project, we were interested in finding out to what extent perceptual or motor deficits in the speech- or language-delayed groups might reflect an overall neurodevelopmental delay. The neurodevelopmental battery included tests of motor control and coordination, balance, tactile and stereognostic perception, and laterality relationships.

Comparison of Normal with Language- and Speech-Delayed Children

Results of the project thus far include comparisons of each separate delayed subject group with the normal control group. These analyses have indicated the following:

Language-delayed children:

1. The language-delayed children as a group were significantly inferior to the normal children on almost all of the tests of auditory identification, sequencing, rapid rate sequencing, and serial memory.

2. The language-delayed children were also significantly inferior to the normal children on some of the tests of visual sequencing, rapid rate sequencing, and serial memory, as well as in cross-modal integration.

3. The language-delayed children were not found to be uniformly delayed on neurodevelopmental subtests. They did, however, show a significantly reduced rate of movement when compared to normal children. This rate of movement deficit extended to gross and fine movements, and to movements of the limbs and of the speech musculature. The language-delayed children did not, however, make a significantly greater number of errors in generating movement sequences, except on a sequenced oral volitional (nonspeech) movement task ($p < .05$).

4. The language-delayed children also showed impairment of tactile perception on the neurodevelopmental battery.

5. The language-delayed children did not show greater difficulty than the normal children on tests of balance, nor were there differences in laterality.

6. The language-delayed children showed some involuntary movements of the hand and arm when asked to maintain a posture of arms outstretched, hands pronated, with the eyes closed.

Speech-delayed children:

1. The speech-articulation-delayed children were not significantly different from the normal children in their performance on any of the auditory perceptual tests administered; they showed relatively mild difficulties in the visual and tactile modalities, and none in the tests of cross-modal integration.

2. The speech-delayed children did not show a rate-of-movement deficit on the motor control and coordination subtests of the neurodevelopmental battery nor on speech or oral motor tasks. They made a significantly greater number of errors in generating movement patterns on certain subtests of the neurodevelopmental battery, but not on sequenced oral volitional (nonspeech) tests.

3. The speech-delayed children also showed some involuntary movements when asked to maintain an outstretched posture of hand and arms.

4. These children were heavier and taller than the normal children.

Discrimination of Speech- and Language-Delayed Children from Normal Children

Discriminant function analysis were subsequently carried out for each impaired subject group separately in comparison with the normal group. Discriminant function analysis is a stepwise statistical procedure which is designed to determine that linear combination of variables which best discriminates subject groups from one another. Variables are tested sequentially, one at a time, for their ability to increase significantly the precision of classification. A classification matrix is prepared and examined at each step so that the effect of inclusion of each new variable can be estimated. The analyses were carried out in stages. Only those variables that were significantly different for the delayed and the normal groups in univariate comparisons, or that were considered to be biologically important, were included. First the analyses were performed separately for different classes of variables (e.g., for demographic, neurodevelopmental, auditory perceptual, and other variables).

A final composite discriminant function was then computed with all variables that were found to be significant in the series of equations computed for individual variable classes. It should be observed that variables that were highly significant in univariate analysis might not contribute to the precision of classification in the presence of other predictor variables. They might be preempted from the resulting equation by other variables with which they were highly correlated.

The variables that were found to contribute most significantly to the discrimination between normal and language-delayed children were, in order of importance:

1. Rapid Word Production subtest (speech motor battery)
2. Cross-modal Rapid Rate Sequencing subtest (sequencing of tone and light flash)

3. Identification of synthetic consonant–vowel syllables (/ba/ versus /da/)
4. Double Simultaneous Tactile Stimulation subtest (neurodevelopmental battery)
5. Visual Rapid Rate Sequencing subtest (sequencing of nonsense shapes)
6. Two-Finger Identification subtest (neurodevelopmental battery)

A classification matrix derived from this discriminant function analysis is shown in Table 3.1. It will be observed that 97% of the subjects in the two groups, that is, all of the normal children and all but two of the language-delayed children, were correctly classified by the equation representing these six variables.

For the articulation-impaired and normal children a different set of vari-

TABLE 3.1

Discriminant Analysis for Normal and Language-Delayed Children: Variables Entering the
Discriminant Function Equation and the Resulting Classification Matrix

Summary table Step number	Variable entered and removed	F value to enter or remove	P value	Number of variables included	Approximate F statistics	df
1	Rapid production of words	50.49	.001	1	50.49	1,57
2	Rapid cross-modal sequencing of tone and light	10.99	.01	2	35.17	2,56
3	Identification of CV syllables /ba/ versus /da/	6.95	.05	3	28.26	3,55
4	Double simultaneous stimulation (face and hand)	7.93	.01	4	25.84	4,54
5	Rapid visual sequencing of "e" and "k" graphemes	10.06	.01	5	26.16	5,53
6	Two-finger identification	4.09	.05	6	23.75	6,52

Classification matrix

Group	Percentage correct	Number of cases classified into group Normal	Language delayed
Normal	100.0	33	0
Language delayed	92.3	2	24
Total	96.6	35	24

TABLE 3.2

Discriminant Analysis for Normal and Speech-Articulation-Delayed Children: Variables Entering the Discriminant Function Equation and the Resulting Classification Matrix

Step number	Variable entered and removed	Summary table F value to enter or remove	P value	Number of variables included	Approximate F statistic	df
1	Weight	14.11	.001	1	14.11	1, 55
2	Rapid visual sequencing of "e" and "k" graphemes	4.83	.05	2	9.96	2, 54
3	Identification of the CV syllables /bae/ versus /dae/	4.52	.05	3	8.58	3, 53

Classification matrix

Group	Percentage correct	Number of cases classified into group	
		Normal	Speech delayed
Normal	80.0	24	6
Speech delayed	77.8	6	21
Total	78.9	30	27

ables was found to contribute to discrimination. These were, in order of importance:

1. Weight
2. Visual rapid rate sequencing of the letters e and k
3. Identification of the synthetic consonant–vowel syllables /bæ/ and /bæ/ (a task on which the performance of the articulation-impaired children was superior)

The classification matrix deriving from this second discrimination function is shown in Table 3.2. It will be observed that 79% of the subjects in the normal and speech-delayed groups were classified correctly (80% of normal children and 78% of the speech-delayed children).

These analyses suggest that certain perceptual and/or motor deficits may be highly characteristic of speech- and/or language-delayed children. Measures of these characteristics might prove useful adjuncts to identification of such children. More importantly, they may describe the clusters of phenotypic expression of speech- and language-related disorders that run in families. Before employing such characteristic deficits as markers in family studies, however, it might be important to find out to what extent they are related to speech or language disorders in children.

Relations between Perceptual and Motor Deficits and Speech and Language Disorders

Multivariate analyses were carried out in the original project in order to test for such relationships. First, a weighted index representing each child's level of functioning in receptive and expressive language was derived from standard test scores (see Stark, Tallal, & Mellits, 1982). A speech articulation score had also been obtained. Second, multivariate analyses were run to determine which variables were most highly correlated with, or predictive of, the weighted speech and language scores. These analyses were carried out separately for the normal and for the speech- and language-delayed groups. Classes of variables (e.g., auditory perceptual variables, visual perceptual variables, speech motor variables, and neurodevelopmental variables) were entered into separate multivariate analyses first. Subsequently, a final composite multivariate analysis was computed, entering only those variables that had made a significant contribution in the multivariate analyses for each separate variable class. A final composite equation was obtained for prediction of the level of each of the language abilities of interest in the three subject groups.

The results obtained were as follows:

1. *Level of receptive language:* Four auditory perceptual variables, taken together, correlated significantly and most highly with level of receptive language in the language-delayed children. These were rapid rate sequencing of the CV syllables /ba/ and /da/, identification of these syllables with 40 msec. consonant-vowel transitions; identification of these syllables with 80 msec consonant–vowel transitions; and identification of 2 complex tones of 250 msec duration (multiple $R = .85$). These variables were also correlated quite highly with receptive language in normal children. In the normal children, however, a quite different set of variables related to reading ability were found to be *most* highly correlated with level of receptive language (multiple $R = .94$).

2. *Level of expressive language:* The variable measuring the number of speech sounds (phonemes) in error, correlated most highly with level of expressive language in the language-delayed children (multiple $R = .74$). A timed visual cancellation or marking subtest (marking the letters *en* in real words) and sequencing of the consonant–vowel syllables /bæ/ and /dæ/ also contributed significantly to "prediction" of level of expressive language in these children (multiple R for all three variables taken together $= .89$). In the normal children, variables that were related to reading—namely, scores on an auditory sequencing task in which the children had to sequence six different syllables, and a visual serial memory variable (memory for two nonsense figures presented in sets of four at a time)—when taken together, contributed most significantly to level of expressive language (multiple $R = .94$).

The results reported under (1) and (2) support the growing conviction among investigators that receptive and expressive language have quite different bases and developmental processes (Chapman, 1981).

3. *Speech articulation ability*

a. Rate of syllable production variables, that is, rate and accuracy of artic-ulatory movement in producing syllables (speech motor battery) contributed most highly to prediction of speech articulation ability in *language-delayed* children (multiple $R = .86$).

b. Prediction of speech articulation in the *normal children* may be less meaningful as few of them made *any* errors, or even developmental misar-ticulations, and thus the spread of scores was small. However, a number of variables were found to correlate highly with speech articulation ability in these normal children. These were, in order of importance, identification of high and low tones (250 msec in duration), a test of graphesthesia on the surface of the palm (neurodevelopmental battery), a cross-modal rapid rate sequencing sub-test, and a right–left discrimination task (neurodevelopmental battery; multiple $R = .92$).

c. In the *speech-articulation-delayed* children, neurodevelopmental vari-ables contributed most to prediction of speech articulation scores. These vari-ables were duration of involuntary movements on a hand–arm posturing task, errors in sequencing thumb–finger opposition movements with the right hand, and errors in the finger-to-nose task for the right hand (multiple $R = .76$). The demographic variables of family history of speech and language problems together with a history of delayed motor development in the subjects them-selves also contributed to this prediction.

Thus, the findings suggest that the nature of articulation problems in chil-dren who do and in children who do not have receptive or expressive language problems may be somewhat different. The findings also indicate that perceptual and motor deficits are related to level of speech and language ability in the delayed children. However, the nature of the relationships between perceptual and motor deficits and language disorders in children remains unclear. They are not necessarily causal relationships. The present findings do not indicate that there is an inherent difference in the basic functioning of the perceptual or motor systems in language-delayed and normal children. Instead, it seems likely that perceptual and/or motor learning may be delayed in children with speech and language disorders.

These delays in perceptual and motor learning, and also the speech and language deficits with which they are correlated, may be related in turn to a common factor or factors not dealt with in our investigation. It may be possible for some language-delayed children eventually to overcome these delays by employing compensatory or alternative language-learning strategies. Moreover, the language-delayed children may, with maturity, show gains with respect to perceptual and motor skills, just as they show gains in verbal abilities.

CONCLUSIONS

The approaches to identification and classification that were used in the study that has been described may not be entirely appropriate for the purposes of genetic studies. However, the findings suggest that the identification of speech- and language-delayed children through both the judgment of parents, teachers, and clinicians, and the use of standardized measures of speech and language, is more reliable than identification through either one of these approaches alone. Even so, in the ascertainment of index cases in family studies, it may be advisable to concentrate upon language-impaired children who are at least 7–8 years of age. Children identified as having significant speech or language disorders at these older ages are unlikely to show significant improvement or to catch up with their peers.

Speech and language disorders should also be defined in relation to cognitive functioning. This is not to say that they must be defined by exclusion, that is, as disorders that occur in the absence of mental retardation. Instead, it is important to consider that, even in a child in the mild to moderate range of mental retardation, language disorders may be indicated wherever verbal abilities are significantly lower than nonverbal abilities.

It may also be the case that the efforts to identify subtypes of speech and language disorders, although important to studies of the etiology of these disorders, may not be meaningful in genetic studies. Subtypes may be found to represent the same defect at the gene level.

Measures of language-related perceptual and motor skills may not be useful for the purpose of initial identification of index cases in genetic or family studies of speech and language disorders. These measures may describe variation within some particular population quite sensitively, and yet be improper tools for discriminating accurately and reliably between normal children and children with different speech and language pathologies. At the same time, such measures of perceptual and motor abilities may suggest differences in localization of dysgenesis or lesion within the central nervous system which may be reflected in different subtypes of speech and language disorder. They may also serve as useful markers for speech and language disorders in family studies. In other words, the relatives of language-disordered children who present isolated perceptual and motor deficits or a history of such deficits in childhood may carry the particular gene for speech and language disorders without experiencing the abnormal effects of that gene to the fullest extent.

There is at present no readily available means to address directly the underlying etiology of speech and language disorders. It may well be that family studies, combined with the use of standard intelligence tests and speech and language tests and also with measures of perceptual and motor abilities, may offer the most powerful tools for defining homogeneous phenotypic entities and enabling us to begin to study these entities.

REFERENCES

Allen, D. V., & Bliss, L. S. *Evaluation of procedures for screening preschool children for signs of impaired language development.* Second Interim Report, Contract NS 6 2353, NINCDS. Bethesda, Md.: Department of Health, Education and Welfare, 1979.

Brown, R., Cazden, C., & Bellugi, U. The child's grammar from I to III. *Psycholinguistics: Selected papers by Roger Brown.* New York: Free Press, 1970.

Chapman, R. Cognitive development and language comprehension in 10 to 21 month olds. In R. E. Stark (Ed.), *Language behavior in infancy and early childhood.* Amsterdam: Elsevier–North Holland, 1981.

Ingram, D. Early patterns of grammatical development. In R. E. Stark (Ed.) *Language behavior in infancy and early childhood.* Amsterdam: Elsevier-North Holland, 1981.

Marge, M. The general problem of language disabilities in children. In J. V. Irwin & M. Marge (Eds.), *Principles of childhood language disabilities.* New York: Appleton-Century-Crofts, 1972.

Morley, M. E. *The development and disorders of speech in childhood* (2nd ed.). London: Livingstone, 1965.

Nelson, K. Structure and strategy in learning to talk. Monographs of the Society for Research in Child Development Vol. 38 (Serial no 149), 1973.

Nelson, K. E. Language-learning styles that combine semantic, syntactic and discourse elements. Paper presented at the Second International Congress for the Study of Child Language. Vancouver, British Columbia, 1981.

Stark, R. E., & Tallal, P. Perceptual and motor deficits in language impaired children. In R. W. Keith (Ed.), *Central auditory and language disorders in children.* Houston: College Hill Press, 1980.

Stark, R. E., & Tallal, P. Selection of children with specific language impairment. *Journal of Speech and Hearing Disorders,* 1981, *46,* 114–122.

Stark, R. E., Tallal, P., & Mellits, E. D. Quantification of language abilities in children. In N. Lass (Ed.), *Speech and language: Advances in basic research and practice* (Vol. 7). New York: Academic Press, 1982.

Wechsler, D. Wechsler Preschool and Primary Scale of Intelligence. New York: The Psychological Corporation, 1963.

Wechsler, D. Wechsler Intelligence Scale for Children–Revised. New York: The Psychological Corporation, 1974.

4

Physiological Specification of the Phenotype in Genetic Language Disorders: Prospects for the Use of Indicators of Localized Brain Metabolism[1]

FRANK WOOD
REBECCA FELTON

INTRODUCTION

Technological pioneering in brain-imaging techniques has in the last 2 decades progressed to the point of enabling—within certain limits of temporal and spatial resolution—the measurement and imaging of localized processes believed to reflect functional neuronal activity in the normal, working human brain. Simultaneously, as this volume so richly attests, there have been truly remarkable advances in the understanding and characterization of genetic factors responsible for disorders of language processing in children and adults. Our purpose in this chapter is to consider the overlapping of these two lines of development. This overlapping has all the perils and possibilities that attend any meeting of two pioneering expeditions. Can they help each other chart the wilderness? Or, will they exchange ritual pleasantries and go their separate ways, each to conquer their own manifestly destined territory? It requires only minimal insight to see that the latter alternative too often characterizes the contemporary state of affairs in the neurosciences, to say nothing of the larger realm of the biological and social sciences. On the other hand, that state of affairs makes the current work of integration and synthesis relatively easy: It is the simple, first steps which are now needed—the sort of steps that come from straightforward sharing of perspectives and the consequent broadening of the overall view.

The specifics of the topic dictate the considerations that must be raised in this chapter. We must ask whether these new technologies can help in any

[1]Supported in part by Grant #NIH-NINCDS-5-POINS-06655 from the United States Public Health Service.

GENETIC ASPECTS OF
SPEECH AND LANGUAGE DISORDERS

significant way to define normal and abnormal language processes. At the same time, we must consider whether the specifics of normal or disordered language, arising from genetic or other factors, impose special methodological requirements on the use of these new technologies. At this quite preliminary stage we must, moreover, limit ourselves to the most obvious methodological issues: The data at this stage offer little more than hints of hypotheses. Accordingly, we will first of all, and for the bulk of this chapter, consider methodological requirements and limitations for the use of localized indicators of brain metabolism in characterizing normal and disordered language. Next, and more briefly, we will consider some of the special limitations imposed by the genetic aspects of the inquiry.

SPECIFIC METHODOLOGICAL QUESTIONS

The Limits of Resolution: Space, Time, and Complexity

The variety of techniques for characterizing local brain activity differ in their resolution in the domains of time, space, and complexity. Spatial resolution refers to the two- or three-dimensional brain geography and to the question of how small a region can be separately characterized as functionally distinct from an adjacent region of similar size. Temporal resolution refers to the time across which the localized metabolic activity is measured or indexed. Complexity resolution refers to the total number of independent sites whose local functional metabolic activity can be simultaneously but individually measured. We further define complexity resolution as an inverted U-shaped function of the number of such sites, so that when their number exceeds a certain critical level the result is said to lack complexity resolution in the specific sense that the number of data points substantially exceeds the channel capacity of the observer. Without unifying algorithms of some sort to "chunk" or impose patterning on the set of data points, the observer sees *fewer,* not more, "events" in the mass of data points.

Electrophysiological techniques, using external electrodes, are a class of techniques sharing some similarities with but not actually belonging to the class of techniques under consideration in this chapter. That is partly because their spatial resolution is extremely coarse, permitting only very crude and approximate localizations within the brain, but it is mainly because of the indirect and uncertain relationship between functional neuronal activity and the externally measured EEG signal. Nonetheless, these techniques have been highly instructive in brain–behavior research, and some of their specific features of resolution are worth noting, for the sake of comparison with the techniques to be considered here. Electrophysiological techniques are extremely fine in their temporal resolution, down to the order of milliseconds. The measurement situation, therefore, always involves an extended time course, during which the measurements at a given site change rapidly. This yields a highly resolute and rich temporal record, making it especially suitable for measurement of the impact of finely and carefully specified independent variables, an impact whose unfolding time· course can be delineated with great precision. The issues of complexity resolution tend, as well, to devolve mostly into this time domain, where a variety of multivariate procedures have been developed for reducing the complexities of the temporal sequence of data points. Still, interlocational effects, such as cross-correlation functions, are also beginning to be appreciated in this research literature, leading to the development of some techniques for simplifying the geographical domain as well.

The regional cerebral blood flow technique is the oldest of the methods for measuring localized brain activity. It depends for its validity upon the tight coupling, at least in normals, between regional cerebral blood flow and oxidative metabolism, and this coupling is generally accepted (Raichle, Grubb, Gado, Eichling, & Ter-Pogossian, 1976). Regional cerebral blood flow can actually be measured either by the use of external scintillation detectors to monitor the clearance of radioactive xenon or by the use of positron emission tomography itself. For the present purpose of comparing spatial, temporal, and complexity resolution across methods, we consider the 133-xenon inhalation method—the only blood flow method to have been widely used with normals, so far. This method has spatial resolution only in two dimensions, around the cortical surface, just underneath the external skull. It "observes" circles on the cortex of approximately 2 or 3 cm in diameter, and usually employs between 16 and 32 separate detectors, hence that number of "circles" on cortex. More specifically, the technique isolates gray matter in and just beneath the circles of resolution, and this feature makes it particularly interesting for the investigation of functional neuronal activity. The temporal resolution—in the sense of the length of time over which the underlying activity is summed—is technically 11 min. However, the gray matter flow is disproportionately determined by the first 3 or 4 min, and a given state or activity of brain can sometimes be sustained for just that length of time, and valid estimates obtained. As there is only a single, summed value for a given time period, all of the complexity is invested in the spatial domain. The number of simultaneous detectors facilitates not only visual inspection but also a variety of multivariate procedures to characterize relationships between sites and across subjects.

Positron emission tomography, when used to assess localized glucose utilization in the brain, has much higher spatial resolution—easily less than a centimeter, and that in three dimensional "slices" through the brain volume. The temporal resolution, however, is less favorable: It takes on the order of 30–40 min to obtain an adequate summation of activity. The scan therefore reflects the total metabolic activity of each region summed across 30 or 40 min. Any state or activity of the brain must therefore be maintained and held constant across that time period. Again, as there is only one datum in the time domain, all of the complexity is in the spatial domain. The number of separate sites or "pixels" is well into the hundreds or thousands, far in excess of what can be managed without a pattern recognition procedure. The obvious procedure is to arrange the pixels in a one-to-one mapping of reconstructed brain slices, and to examine the set of slices visually. This recruits normal human visual pattern perception processes, including contour enhancement, figure—ground differentiation, and the like, thus highlighting the visually salient features of the data set. At the same time, the very act of examining the scans visually necessarily obscures relationships that may exist between spatially remote regions of the brain. Elementary neuroanatomy helps in this regard, so that one is prone to notice, for example, the simultaneous occurrence of high right-thalamic and right-parietal metabolism, but as such observations depend on existing knowledge of functional neuroanatomy, hitherto unrecognized relationships between distant regions may still escape notice.

Nuclear magnetic resonance can in principle be employed to assess localized metabolism, through electromagnetic indices of localized phosphorous turnover. Although current techniques limit the spatial volume resolution to something on the order of 10 cm^3, with temporal resolution in the 5–10 min range, it is possible that further developments may enable much greater spatial resolution. The same issues of complexity resolution would apply here as apply in the case of positron emission tomography.

Two broader issues apply to the question of resolution. The first has to do with the upper limits of complexity resolution. If we permit ourselves to speculate about developments well into the future, we soon realize that successive hierarchies of pattern recognition algorithms, applied to ever more temporally and spatially resolute data, could finally result in a structure whose complexity approached that of the brain itself. We would then encounter the classical paradox of self-reference in formal systems, in this case the paradox of the brain understanding itself. Although we may consider ourselves far, far away from that level of complexity, we are certainly far enough along that we must begin to ask whether the interpretive algorithms we apply are not themselves examples of the phenomena we wish to study. At a minimum, it behooves us to recognize the particular biasing that attends some interpretive algorithm—as is already apparent when we rely on visual inspection of positron emission tomography scans.

The second consideration derives from the first: Scientific progress often depends precisely on coarser rather than finer measurement instruments. If the ultimate characterization of the brain would require accounting for each of the 10^{14} synapses it contains, then progress would be a long time in coming. It takes only a single example—the theory of evolution—to remind us that progress sometimes involves looking at larger rather than smaller units of space and time. The summation of the activity of large, geographically contiguous populations of neurons across substantial intervals of time provides a much coarser analysis than would be provided, for example, by single cell recordings from each of the participating neurons. To the extent that brain activity does become spatially and temporally concentrated—differentially so across time and across brain geography—this summation is favorable for fundamental advance in then the neurosciences. It is ultimately an empirical question how much of brain activity can be reliably and validly described with these coarse summations. Existing data suggest that many phenomena, including many aspects of language processing, do map onto these coarser units of brain space and time.

Experimental Design: The Isolation of Specific Language Processing

How can we isolate language itself as the specific process being measured with these localized indicators of brain metabolism? The classical answer is: by engaging subjects in a language task and measuring localized blood flow or metabolism during that task, and comparing those results to the ones obtained during the execution of a carefully specified control task. Indeed, this method, using large enough groups of normal subjects, is indispensable to research in brain–behavior relations. However, there are a number of complexities which threaten to contaminate if not utterly spoil the concept of a "pure" experimental comparison. Some of these complexities have to do with data analysis, and are considered in the next section of this chapter. Here we consider only those complexities associated with the construction of a suitable experimental design.

The first problem is in the precision with which the control condition is specified. Different problems arise at different degrees of precision of the experimental versus control difference. At one extreme, one could compare some language task to a quiet, eyes-closed, resting base line measurement. In that case, the comparison is obviously impure, as the experimental condition differs from the resting base line in many more ways than language alone. If the language task consisted of listening to a story, for example, with the knowledge that comprehension would later be tested, then auditory stimulation itself—irrespective of its verbal qualities—would be an obvious confound. Moreover, the resting base line is a less well-controlled state than the story-listening task: Subjects may have varied widely in their covert mental processes during the resting base line, with corresponding variance in their brain activity and in their localized metabolic "landscapes." That much is obvious. However, there are also obvious problems at the other extreme of "purity" of experimental versus control comparison. What is, after all, a suitable control for listening to a story? Shall it be listening to a musical passage? That leaves speech sounds as one of several obvious confounds. Shall it be listening to the story, but doing so in the expectation of later being asked to recognize specific words from the story? If so, how can the subject in the control condition be prevented from actually listening to and understanding the story?

A more specific problem is that in attempting a refined experimental versus control comparison we naturally end up (essentially by definition) manipulating only some subprocess of language. In this case, even if we assume that the manipulation is successful in inducing two different states in the subjects (one having to do with the active listening to the story, the other having to do with the active listening for specific words apart from the story line), some features of language itself are shared across the two conditions. The local metabolic response associated with those shared features of language processing cannot, therefore, be characterized in such an experiment. That also raises the associated question of whether the manipulation of the particular subprocess of language (in this case listening to a story) results only in a "language" difference. Could it not be, for example, that listening to a story evokes visual imagery, and that it is the visual imagery that is responsible for the local metabolic differences in the two conditions?

The point of all this is not just the difficulty of specifying an adequate control for a complex language task—that is a difficulty inherent in any type of psycholinguistic research. However, complexities of this type, which can be termed difficulties in the construct validation of any single experimental design, are less damaging in a research paradigm that is well established, replete with converging operations, replications, and the like. In this case, as we are in the earliest and most primitive stages of the use of localized indicators of metabolism for studying behavioral processes in general, to say nothing of language processes in particular, these complexities are still quite dangerous. The only escape from them is to avoid premature conclusions and to await the emergence of converging and replicative studies.

A second major difficulty with carefully controlled experiments has to do with the sensitivity of the brain activity measurement techniques. As a given experimental versus control comparison is made more refined and subtle, its impact on gross, localized brain metabolism may become equally subtle. In such cases, the effects may be swamped by incidental differences in task difficulty, intrinsic or extrinsic reward value of the tasks, arousal and attentional factors, and similar variables. The effects of such variables on brain activity during language tasks has already been shown (see Halsey, Blauenstein, Wilson, & Wills, 1980a; Risberg, Halsey, Wills, & Wilson, 1975; Wood, Stump, McKeehan, Sheldon, & Proctor, 1980, respectively, for difficulty, extrinsic reward, and pharmacological dearousal).

Studies of language activation illustrate these problems, and some of them are clearly worth reviewing. The first, historic study of lateralized and localized brain activation, in response to a language task, was done by Risberg, Halsey, Wills, and Wilson (1975). Normal volunteers engaged either in problems requiring the solution of verbal analogies or in problems requiring perceptual closure. In one condition, subjects were well paid for accurate performance whereas in the other condition they were not. Under reward conditions, the verbal task engendered significant left-posterior hemisphere increases compared to the resting base line; whereas the perceptual closure task produced a broader (frontal as well as parietal) increase in the right hemisphere. Under conditions of no reward, the increases were in the same direction but were not statistically significant.

Technically, the relevant independent variable is a combination of either of two modality-specific tasks (verbal analogies and perceptual closure) with high reward, with both combinations being compared to a resting base line. Given that some sort of laterality effect has been clearly demonstrated, one could certainly argue that it is the effort or response to the reward contingency which is lateralized, rather than the verbal versus visual–spatial processing itself. The experiment, standing alone, could not refute that interpretation. Somewhat further along the continuum of experimental refinement, Knopman, Rubens, Klassen, Meyer, and Niccum (1980) compared a verbal and a nonverbal auditory task. The verbal task consisted of listening to a list of nouns, and signaling whenever one of them was "something to eat" whereas the nonverbal tasks consisted of listening to pairs of half-second white noise bursts, signaling in each case which member of the pair was the softer. Compared to the resting base line, both the verbal and the nonverbal tasks produced focal left Wernicke's area increases. These results are quite challenging and should provoke further research to test a variety of possible explanations. Perhaps any classification or categorizing task, as it is by definition analytic, is therefore a left-hemisphere task, so that in a certain sense both tasks were "verbal" tasks. On the other hand, for all we know from this experiment, any auditory processing may be lateralized to the left hemisphere. Thus, the experiment illustrates how early experiments, at least in this particular field, serve mainly to broaden rather than narrow the theoretical possibilities.

Granted the sort of complexities that have been illustrated, we may nevertheless ask whether existing studies have begun to result in any sort of converging evidence as to the nature of localized brain activation in normal versus pathological language processing. In answering such a question, it is feasible to review just the inhalation regional cerebral blood flow literature, as the injection method of blood flow measurement is only unilateral, and as positron emission tomography does not yet have enough normal or language-disordered cases, subjected to careful experimental control, to permit us to draw conclusions. The conclusions regarding normal versus pathological language that can be provisionally entertained from the inhalation regional cerebral blood flow literature can be summarized as follows:

1. It has been difficult to show strong focal activation in the left hemisphere, with conventional language tasks, in normal subjects. See the studies already cited, as well as Wood, Taylor, Penny, and Stump (1980), in which a semantic categorizing task elicited only small increases; Gur and Reivich (1980), in which a verbal analogies task did elicit focal left-temporal increases, but increases that were rather highly variable, not only in the focal area, but in other left-hemisphere areas as well. At least some left hemisphere increases, referable at least in part to specific language processing, are usually shown with

verbal tasks. Both the sheer quantity of those increases and their extent (focal versus diffuse) are at present not systematically related to their independent variables, so that they are still difficult to predict. The full range of language processes, from simplest to most complex, has not even been sampled in the extant studies, must less systematically explored.

2. Aphasics, stutterers, and one patient with alexia without agraphia have tended to show higher than normal levels of regional cerebral blood flow, when engaged in language tasks challenging their particular disability. These increases have tended to be bilateral and often hyperfrontal. See Halsey, Blauenstein, Wilson, and Wills (1980a, 1980b) and Wood, Stump, McKeehan, Sheldon, and Proctor (1980). In cases of this type, especially when the lesions are small and chronic, the relatively coarse spatial resolution of the inhalation regional cerebral blood flow technique will often completely obscure the actual lesion, leaving the diffuse flow increases as the prominent features of the cortical flow landscapes of such patients during attempted language processing.

The bilaterally diffuse character of these increases argues against interpreting them as indicative of the operation of specific compensatory brain mechanisms. The correct explanation for these generalized increases has not been established. In such cases, where many explanations are possible, the simplest one may be the most preferable on grounds of parsimony and heuristic utility. In this case, we can therefore provisionally entertain the simple explanation: When a focal lesion renders a certain language process difficult or impossible, then the attempt to engage that process is arousing and stimulative of diffuse cortical activation.

It is instructive to compare the above phenomenon to its converse: the challenging of aphasic patients by nonspecific, multimodal, unselective stimulation (Meyer, Sakai, Yamaguchi, Yamamoto, & Shaw, 1980). This multiple psychophysiological activation, as these investigators term it, involves a continuous delivery of constantly changing auditory and visual stimulation, with frequent demands for all sorts of responses—such as counting, answering questions, looking at objects, visualizing certain things, and making certain hand movements. In normals this procedure results in diffuse, bilateral increases in flow. When applied to aphasic patients, however, it induces those flow increases only in the right hemisphere. There is marked attenuation of the flow increases in the left hemisphere, the more so in the most impaired patients. Opting again for the simplest explanation, we may suppose that when aphasic patients confront a nonspecific stimulus barrage, they will select and respond to those features of the barrage that engage right- but not left-hemisphere functioning. The data thus create an interesting dissociation. When a task requires selective attention to language, aphasics will respond to it in the same way that normals respond to nonspecific, nonselective tasks—with diffuse, bilateral arousal and activation of cortical mechanisms. When aphasics are confronted by a nonspecific and nonselective task, they will respond the same way normals do if confronted by a task demanding selective spatial activation—with unilateral right-hemisphere flow increases. It is also worth noting that this phenomenon arises only under conditions of behavioral challenge, not under the relatively relaxed conditions of a resting base line.

Statistical Properties: Distributions, Variances, and Correlations

In common with many other physiological measurement situations, regional cerebral blood flow techniques often yield positively skewed distributions across a sample of normal subjects. (There are not yet enough normal groups of sufficient size to permit this conclusion with respect to positron emission tomography.) That skewing may reflect no more than the physiological "floor" of the measurements. However, it is interesting that sometimes the skewing is so pronounced as to result in a frank bimodality of the flow values, so that one is lead to suspect a typology of subjects or of strategies chosen by subjects, resulting in the bimodal distributions. In some studies the bimodality is simply present in the raw data but not remarked upon (Wood, 1983), but at least in one case these subject variables have been formally studied and their highly significant effect shown (Gur, Gur, Obrist, Hungerbuhler, Younkin, Rosen, Skolnick & Reivich, 1982). In this study, handedness and sex were each shown to have statistically independent as well as interacting effects on hemispheric blood flow under resting base line, verbal activation, and spatial activation conditions.

That handedness and sex should be among the subject variables that explain bimodalities or multimodalities in the distributions of flow values across subjects naturally gives confidence to a program of genetic research in this area. At the same time, it stimulates us to be all the more cautious in the use of any group of subjects, or in the use of means as accurate estimates of the performance of those groups. Highly theoretically important subject variables are all too easy to overlook, unless close attention is given to the shapes of the distributions.

Another aspect of the distributions of flow values is the fact that their variances are often correlated with their means. One of us (Wood, 1983) has argued this point extensively elsewhere, suggesting that a high variance coupled with a high mean can be considered indicative of a situation of disinhibition or disregulation. For example, if verbal activation produces focal left-temporal mean increases, but also a proportional increase in variance, then the verbal activation may be considered disinhibitory, in the sense that subjects are freer under that condition. They show a greater variety of flow values at that particular site than they are able to show in the resting base line, or in an alternative spatial activation state. At a minimum, the statistical properties of the impact of the verbal activation on the left-temporal lobe are not those we would expect from an activation which constrains or excites that area to some statistically similar extent across subjects. Conventional parametric statistical procedures are accordingly risky, and it is not enough to rely on the general robustness of such procedures to violations of the assumption of homogeneity of variance. Nor is it suitable, in the long range, to transform the variables so as to eliminate the nonnormality and inhomogeneity of variance, as doing so would obscure the very subject differences generating those nonnormalities and greater variances. Indeed, when the means and variances are explicitly considered and statistically analyzed in their own right, radically different conclusions can emerge. For example, in reanalyzing the Gur and Reivich (1980) study mentioned earlier, Wood (1983) came to almost the opposite conclusion from that originally proposed by the authors. On the basis of an analysis of the correlation of means and variances within hemispheres, Wood proposed that the verbal activation condition was relatively *non*activated, compared to both the resting base line and the spatial activation condition, both of which were considered to reflect an excitatory type of behavioral activation.

Granted the complexities of interpretation of the variance of flow values, it is nevertheless instructive to examine the correlations of a given set of flow values with either another set of flow values or an external behavioral criterion. Nonparametric correlations can be employed when necessary. There have been only a few studies using correlations with task accuracy, but in every case they have been quite instructive. In the same Gur and Reivich (1980) study, the strength of the hemispheric asymmetry in favor of right-hemisphere activation was found to correlate with the accuracy of performance on the spatial task. Thus, in contrast to some other situations where higher flow suggests greater difficulty in task execution, this correlation suggests that higher right-hemisphere flow is indeed relevant to better task performance. Especially interesting are two studies showing inverse correlations with task accuracy (Wood, Taylor, Penny, & Stump, 1980; Leli, Hannay, Falgout, Wilson, Wills, Katholi, & Halsey, 1982). In the former study, recognition memory accuracy, for auditorily presented words was found to be highly inversely correlated with left-posterior and bilateral occipital flow. In the latter, a task of right–left discrimination of body parts showed greater suppression of left-posterior flow with greater task accuracy. A variety of interpretations are possible (see Wood, 1983). For purposes of the present discussion, it is enough simply to note that much additional information can be gained by correlating flow or metabolism values with accuracy of task performance, and potentially with other aspects of task performance (such as speed).

Correlations between flow measurements at different brain sites have been even less common and less systematic in the literature. The principal use, so far, has been with homologous left- and right-hemisphere sites. High correlations between homologous probes have been taken as evidence of the absence of lateralized asymmetries in cognitive processing, for example, in peri-Rolandic, sensory motor cortex. Low homologous probe correlations, in contrast, have been taken as indications of lateralized higher functions, often in temporal-parietal association cortex (Prohovnik, Hakansson, & Risberg, 1980; Wood, Taylor, Penny, & Stump, 1980). A fuller exploration of the entire intercorrelation matrix, among all brain sites, would perhaps reveal separate factors, which might change under various conditions of behavioral activation, reflecting the operation of discrete functional systems in the brain. (See Wood, 1983, for a fuller review of this issue.)

GENETIC ISSUES

In considering the issue of how specifically genetic factors may be assessed with indicators of localized brain metabolism, we can initially restrict the question as follows. The specific issue is whether a multichannel measurement of localized brain activity can clarify a genetically based language disorder. Thus, we concern ourselves only with a multichannel measurement, across enough different brain regions to permit distinctive patterns to be observed. We should hardly consider measurements involving only a few or even a single channel, as such measurements would completely eliminate whatever power exists in these techniques for indexing local brain metabolism. By definition, then, the issue before us involves patterns of response across several brain regions, not absolute levels of response in any single brain region.

This qualification presupposes another, more basic one, discussed more extensively earlier. As it is language disorders that are our concern, we limit the question to multichannel brain activity *associated with* or *responsive to* language behavior. We are not asking, therefore, whether a lesion—congenital or otherwise—gives rise to both a language disorder and a physiological abnormality, so that the physiological abnormality is simply a correlate or marker of the language disorder. We ask if there is a specific abnormality in the physiological response to language challenge. Thus, we presume that measurements of localized brain activity may disclose something more basic about the neurobehavioral mechanism of genetically disordered language—more basic, that is, than the final behavioral expression itself.

Thus qualified, we may consider the genetic issues topically, as follows.

Genetic Impact on Distributions and Their Parameters: Discontinuity and Inhomogenous Variance

Except where the genetic determination is highly polygenic (and to that extent essentially part of the normally distributed population variance), the genetic impact on language disorder should cause some segregation and discontinuity from normals. To use an analogy, true dwarfism is rare and its genetic causes (though possibly still polygenic in some cases) are relatively circumscribed. True dwarfism is therefore not continuous with the normal distribution of height in the population, as the latter is the result of a wide range of genetic and environmental influences. The extreme of "normal" short stature is not the same as dwarfism.

The prospect of a discontinuity between genetically determined language disorders and the more normal variation in language skills characteristic of the population at large is theoretically plausible, and even necessary at least to some extent, but the prospect also has an empirical outcome associated with it. If some discontinuity is assumed, at least at the level of the genotype, then we would expect the phenotypic expressions of the genotype to be more variable, more overlapping with normal variance, and less distinct from the normal population—all in proportion to the "distance" between the genotype and its phenotypic expression. The further that "distance," the more chance there is for environmental and other factors to modify it and blur the distinction from normals. Viewed in this light, we naturally expect the behavioral expression (the measured language disorder itself) to be the most subject to this intervening modulation of the genotype. If so, then the measurement of localized brain metabolism in response to language tasks affords the prospect of a somewhat less variable phenotypic manifestation, one that may be a little bit "closer" to the underlying genotype.

Research strategies for identifying this underlying discontinuity, at whatever level it may appear, will inevitably bias the outcome somewhat. Thus, one approach might be simply to take behaviorally extreme individuals, and go backward to physiological and genetic correlates. That procedure would truncate the expected variance among behavioral phenotypes, notwithstanding their common genotype. On the other hand, to identify a genetically extreme and "pure" group, manifestly distinct from the normal population, will not produce such a pure behavioral phenotype, and the characterization of the phenotype by physiological means—localized indicators of brain metabolism in response to language activation—may also be unexpectedly variable, as the physiological mechanisms are also some distance from the genotype and are also subject to many environmental variables.

This problem is made considerably more intricate if it is assumed that language disorder is only one of the probabilistic expressions of the underlying genotype (see Geschwind, Chapter 2, this volume). If it is only an embryonic suppression of certain left-hemisphere maturation and cell migration processes, and if this is in turn only an expression of a more generalized metabolic variant, then we cannot expect language disorders themselves to breed true. In that case, the physiological as well as behavioral characterizations of the phenotype will be *more* variable in the proband sample than in the normal population. If, on the other hand, we regard some subtypes of language disorder as themselves genotypic, hence breeding true, then we should expect at least equal variance, and probably *lower* variance, in the proband sample compared to the normal population (see Finucci & Childs, Chapter 11, this volume). Empirically, then, we can expect the variance of metabolic levels and patterns across subjects to be one of the most important characteristics of these measurements. Examination of those variances will help determine the nature of the correspondence between the genotype and its phenotypic behavioral expression.

Time Course of the Phenotypic Abnormality

There are several trends that occur in the evolution of genetically based language disorders. Sometimes, these trends may contradict each other, producing some intricate interactions. First of all, there is the basic principle that a congenital behavioral deficit will express itself more clearly in later childhood, adolescence, and adulthood than in early infancy and the preschool years. Several factors can be responsible for this particular pattern. If a congenital lesion occurs in an area of cortex whose functioning does not usually mature until later childhood years, then it will be in principle impossible to observe a behavioral deficit from this lesion early in life. At a minimum, it is impossible to observe a reading deficit, for example, at age 2 or 3, when almost no normal child can read. At least in such cases, if there is any deficit at all it will be in some other process, which may or may not be related to language, and which may be a correlated expression of the same lesion. More generally, there is the familiar clinical experience of a child who is modestly language delayed, who manages rather well in the preschool and even the early school years, because the social and academic demands do not yet confront his disability. In the later grades, however, as language becomes more and more the vehicle of learning and as higher level uses of language are required, the child's burden increases, the delay becomes more apparent, and the deficit becomes more easily measurable. In other words, we may propose that in these cases children are able for a while to compensate for their deficits, both because the demands are not so severe and because they can offer other skills which will satisfy teachers and parents, but the compensation finally fails to keep the child at an adequate level of overall performance.

The contrasting trend is also sometimes observed, whereby a disproportionately severe impairment seems to characterize the early years, but the child then seems to "outgrow" this severe deficit and to "catch up." Such cases are also not unfamiliar in clinical experience, and they raise the question of an underlying mechanism distinct from that which we have already proposed. We believe, on the basis of our own experience with such children, that the explanation often lies in the fact that the deficit is in a more elementary language function, one that is essential to mastering the mechanics of language in the early years, but one that is actually less burdensome as language processing devolves onto higher levels of intellectual activity. It is as though a compensatory mechanism develops, either through maturation or learning or both. (See Stark, Mellits, and Tallal, Chapter 3 of this volume, for a fuller discussion of these differential time courses.)

Measures of localized brain metabolism in response to language activation may well assist in discriminating these contrasting trends. Extrapolation from the adult literature (reviewed earlier in this chapter) suggests that we should look for altered patterns of regional brain activity, alterations which would differ according to the present severity of the deficit and the availability of compensatory mechanisms. We should be especially alert to cases where a child with only mild to moderate deficit showed a brain response that was rather different from that shown by adults or children in the acute phase of a similar but acquired deficit. There are not yet any formal studies of this question in the literature, but there are some illustrative case examples. We have already reviewed some of the typical findings with language disorders acquired in adulthood. The isolated case examples of language-impaired and dyslexic children (Hagstadius, 1981) have shown a different pattern: relatively focal right-hemisphere increases during reading and language processing. A quite similar finding has been reported by us (Wood, Stump, McKeehan, Sheldon, & Proctor, 1980), showing greater right than left Broca's area activation during attempted reading out loud by stutterers. It is significant that in this study the case of acquired stuttering in a college-age female (from head trauma at age 13) showed a much greater asymmetry of right frontal activation than was shown by the case of congenital stuttering, though both did show the same pattern. We tentatively surmised that congenital lesions have a much greater opportunity to result in reorganization of the relevant brain mechanisms. In this way, a study of indicators of local brain metabolism in response to language activation may help to discriminate congenital and early acquired lesions from lesions arising later in life, even though the behavioral result is identical.

Similar contrasts between congenital and acquired forms of behavioral disorder have been suggested by other studies using techniques for localized measurement of flow or metabolism. For example, certain schizophrenics have repeatedly been shown to exhibit unexpectedly low indications of frontal lobe functioning. However, the acute, acquired model for this psychosis (amphetamine intoxication) shows hyperfrontal blood flow (Risberg, 1980). Similarly, a childhood case of attention deficit disorder with hyperactivity has been reported to show extremely high frontal flows (Hagstadius, 1981), whereas the corresponding pharmacological model (low catecholaminergic arousal) is accompanied by hypofrontal flows (Risberg, 1980).

Arousal and Attention:
Their Interaction with Language Disorder

The first step in competent analysis of language disorders is to distinguish syndromes that are primarily attentional from those that involve frank selective disorders of language processing itself. Many cases of apparent dyslexia, language impairment, and other learning disabilities are actually due to attention deficit disorder. In such cases, pharmacological management through stimulant medication is often helpful. Indeed, using nothing more than subtests on the Wechsler Intelligence Scale for Children—Revised (WISC-R), it is possible (at least in our clinical population) to predict favorable response to stimulant medication, on the basis of the relative levels of the Verbal Comprehension and Freedom from Distractability factors on the WISC-R (Felton & Wood, in press). In our study, the difference score, derived by subtracting the mean Freedom from Distractability subtest score from the mean Verbal Comprehension subtest score, predicted the response to stimulant medication. The more positive this score, implying a selective Freedom from Distractability deficit with preservation of Verbal Comprehension, the greater the likelihood of favorable response to stimulant medication.

The issue is by no means that simple, however: There are many cases where attentional and language-processing deficits seem to overlap and reinforce each other. Moreover, the spectrum of attentional disorders at the other extreme of arousal (putative overarousal in autism, schizophrenia, and related syndromes) is usually associated with a frank, central language-processing disorder. These disorders have often been ascribed to hyperdopaminergic activity, and are sometimes successfully treated by dopamine antagonists such as haloperidol. In turn, fluctuations of the dopaminergic system, from over- to underactivated levels, apparently are reflected in regional cerebral blood flow and perhaps positron emission tomography measurements, particularly in the frontal lobes. It can in fact be plausibly argued that the familiar hyperfrontatility of regional cerberal blood flow, in many conditions of rest and behavioral activation, is dopaminergically mediated. It is, certainly, uniquely responsive to pharmacological agents known to influence dopaminergic activity selectively. If hyperfrontality is indeed dopaminergically mediated, and if there is a dopaminergic component to some of the classical syndromes of disordered arousal and attention, then regional cerebral blood flow and other indicators of localized metabolism may well be able to help untangle the attentional and processing components of language disorder in children and adults with such syndromes. Even if schizophrenia is not considered to be at base a language disorder, autism often is so considered, and the known properties of the hyperfrontal response in regional cerebral blood flow may provide additional information, otherwise unattainable, as to underlying brain mechanisms. As we have already noted, chronic schizophrenics show the opposite effect, namely hypofrontal flows. Thus, we suspect an inverted U-shaped function, in which extreme and chronic overarousal leads again to a lowering of frontal lobe activity, whereas in the intermediate and milder stages it had resulted in excessive frontal activity.

The observation of the nature and extent of the hyperfrontal response, and its alleged mediation by attentional and arousal mechanisms, should provide important control information for the assessment of language processing in children with primary language disorder. Thus, in adult patients with acquired lesions, the attempt to do the task which the lesion has made difficult or impossible results in strongly hyperfrontal flows, whereas in the remitted state we see an attenuation of these hyperfrontal flows (Halsey, Blauenstein, Wilson, & Wills, 1980b). This phenomenon may also have important implications for tracking the course of rehabilitation, not only of acquired lesions, but also of congenital ones.

CONCLUSIONS

Localized indicators of brain metabolism, including regional cerebral blood flow, positron emission tomography, and, potentially, nucelar magnetic resonance, have a constructive role to play in the specification of phenotypic expression in cases of genetically based language disorder. Using a multichannel physiological response, involving several simultaneously measured brain regions, it is possible to assess total functional neuronal activity in response to language activation. This activity can be disordered in an observable way, either by an acquired lesion or a congenital anomaly, and the two types of impairment apparently produce somewhat different types of abnormality. This may lead to the possibility of stricter specification of the type of language disorder, whether congenital or recently acquired, even though the behavioral expressions are similar. A multitude of methodological and statistical issues attend this emerging research possibility, and they suggest the need for caution in drawing conclusions. Nonetheless, the prospects for observing the patterned brain response to normal and disordered language is an exciting one, full of potential for the neurosciences generally and for explorations of behavioral and language genetics in particular.

REFERENCES

Gur, R. C., Gur, R. E., Obrist, W., Hungerbuhler, R., Younkin, D., Rosen, A. D., Skolnick, B. E., & Reivich, M. Sex and handedness differences in cerebral blood flow during rest and cognitive activity. *Stroke*, 1982, *217*, 659–651.
Gur, R. C. & Reivich, M. Cognitive task effects on hemispheric blood flow in humans: Evidence for individual differences in hemispheric activation. *Brain and Language*, 1980, *9*, 78–92.
Hagstadius, S., Risberg, J., & Prohovnik, I. *Regional cerebral blood flow in cases of childhood language and behavioral disorder.* Paper presented at the ninth annual meeting of the International Neuropsychological Society, Atlanta, Georgia, February 1981.
Halsey, J., Blauenstein, U., Wilson, E., & Wills, E. rCBF activation in a patient with right homonymous hemianopia and alexia without agraphia. *Brain and Language*, 1980, *9*, 137–140. (a)
Halsey, J., Blauenstein, U., Wilson, E., & Wills, E. Brain activation in the presence of brain damage. *Brain and Language*, 1980, *9*, 47–60. (b)
Knopman, D. S., Rubens, A. B., Klassen, A. C., Meyer, M. W., & Niccum, N. Regional cerebral blood flow patterns during verbal and nonverbal auditory activation. *Brain and Language*, 1980, *9*, 93–112.

Leli, D. A., Hannay, M. J., Flagout, J. C., Wilson, E. M., Willis, E. L., Katholi, C. R., & Halsey, J. H. Focal changes in cerebral blood flow produced by a test of right–left discrimination. *Brain and Cognition, 1,* 206–223.

Maximilian, V. A., Prohovnik, I., Risberg, J., & Hakansson, K. Regional blood flow changes in the left cerebral hemisphere during word pair learning and recall. *Brain and Language,* 1980, *6,* 22–31.

Meyer, J., Sakai, F., Yamaguchi, F., Yamamoto, M., & Shaw, T. Regional changes in cerebral blood flow during standard behavioral activation in patients with disorders of speech and mentation compared to normal volunteers. *Brain and Language,* 1980, *9,* 61–77.

Nilsson, A., Risberg, J., Johanson, M., & Gustafson, L. Regional changes in cerebral blood flow during haloperidol therapy in patients with paranoid symptoms. *Acta Neurologica Scandinavica,* 1976, *56* (Suppl. 64), 478–479.

Prohovnik, I., Hakansson, K., & Risberg, J. Observations on the functional significance of regional cerebral blood flow in "resting" normal subjects. *Neuropsychologia,* 1980, *18,* 203–217.

Raichle, M., Grubb, R., Gado, M., Eichling, J., & Ter-Pogossian, M. Correlation between regional cerebral blood flow and oxidative metabolism. *Archives of Neurology,* 1976, *33,* 523–526.

Risberg, J. Regional cerebral blood flow measurements by Xe-inhalation: Methodology and applications in neuropsychology and applications in neuropsychology and psychiatry. *Brain and Language,* 1980, *9,* 9–34.

Risberg, J., Halsey, J., Wills, E., & Wilson, E. Hemispheric specialization in normal man studied by bilateral measurements of the regional cerebral blood flow: A study with the 133-xenon technique. *Brain,* 1975, *98,* 511–524.

Risberg, J., Maxmillian, A., & Prohovnik I. Changes of cortical activity patterns during habituation to a reasoning task: A study with 133-Xenon inhalation technique for measurement of regional cerebral blood flow. *Neuropsychologia,* 1977, *15,* 793–798.

Wilkinson, I., Bull, J., DuBolay, G., Marshall, J., Ross-Russell, R., & Symon, L. Regional cerebral blood flow in the normal cerebral hemisphere. *Journal of Neurology, Neurosurgery, and Psychiatry,* 1969, *32,* 367–378.

Wood, F. Laterality of cerebral function: Its investigation by measurement of localized brain activity. In J. Hellige, (Ed.), *Cerebral functional asymmetry: Method and theory.* New York: Praeger, 1983, 380–407.

Wood, F., Stump, D., McKeehan, A., Sheldon, S., and Proctor, J. Regional cerebral blood flow response during stuttering, while on and off haloperidol medication: evidence for inadequate left frontal activation during stuttering. *Brain and Language,* 1980, *9,* 124–131.

Wood, F., Taylor, B., Penny, R., & Stump, D. Regional cerebral blood flow response to recognition memory versus semantic classification tasks. *Brain and Language,* 1980, *9,* 113–112.

5

Definition of the Anatomical Phenotype[1]

ALBERT M. GALABURDA

Speech and language disorders are common accompaniments of mental retardation. Mental retardation does not constitute a unified behavioral phenotype, cannot be traced to a single genotype, and, as expected, does not have as its substrate only one brain phenotype. In fact, mental retardation may be the result of metabolic and endocrine diseases, acquired conditions such as infections, trauma, exposure to toxins, tumor, and stroke in early life, chromosomal abnormalities, cerebral malformations, as well as many progressive and nonprogressive syndromes of uncertain etiology, each producing different changes in the brain. It is not the purpose of this chapter to outline the neuroanatomical characteristics of the different mental retardation syndromes, but rather to review the limited literature on the anatomy of specific learning disorders involving speech and language alone. It is hoped that the better definition of the anatomical phenotype in these disorders will help in the understanding of genetic as well as other biological mechanisms underlying the development of normal and abnormal cerebral lateralization, an issue which appears to be central to learning disability.

Specific learning disorders involving speech and language must involve one or only a few psychological processes such that the general level of intelligence (as measured by standard means) is average. Cases in which educational, social, and psychological factors contribute to speech and language difficulties cannot be included because, although such factors may have defina-

[1]Some of the research reported here was supported by grants from the National Institutes of Health (NS-14018), the National Science Foundation (BNS 77-05674), the Wm. Underwood Co., Inc., the Orton Dyslexia Society, and the Essel Fund.

71

ble effects on the anatomical substrate, it is not possible to specify these at this time.

.The neuroanatomical aspects of the specific learning disorders can be summarized briefly because the literature is not extensive. In general, the brains of children and adults with these disorders have not been readily available for analysis, which is surprising inasmuch as developmental language disorders have been recognized for almost 100 years, including a period early in the century when clinical–anatomical correlations were busily researched. Furthermore, early theories of causation, especially those regarding developmental dyslexia, relied heavily on brain models of reading function derived from the analysis of lesioned brains of patients with acquired reading disorders. Thus, although the angular gyrus was theoretically implicated in developmental dyslexia (Hinshelwood, 1917), lesions in actual brains were not demonstrated. An interesting early theory of causation suggested that there may not be actual lesions but rather an imperfect development of the left angular gyrus (Clairborne, 1906), but again this was never documented anatomically. Anatomical studies became less fashionable, and no evidence exists of further attempts to look at the structure of the brain of dyslexics. The opinion of workers in more recent years is best illustrated by the statement by Critchley (1964) who wrote that "it seems unlikely that any tangible [anatomical] evidence will emerge." However, Critchley goes on to say that "it is clearly desirable that pathological studies should be made and published [p. 80]."

One possible explanation for the scarcity of anatomical demonstrations may relate to the fact that learning disability is not associated with early death and the ready availability of brains for study. The affected patients would simply grow to adulthood and possibly outgrow their symptoms, or simply be forgotten or lost to follow-up. However, it is still surprising that brains did not come to be studied by accident alone. If we believe that developmental dyslexia may be so common as to involve 10% of the population (Critchley, 1964) it appears that consistent anatomical findings, if present, would have emerged even if not looked for. One possibility is that the findings may be consistent yet subtle, and have thus escaped detection. Another possibility is that learning disabilities, and even developmental dyslexia alone, do not constitute a single disorder and may have several anatomical substrates, making the recognition of structure–function relationships difficult. Yet another possibility is that the findings are not altogether amenable to discovery by the routine neuropathological methods. Thus the brain in early Parkinson's disease, for instance, might appear normal in a section that is not stained for melanin pigment. Similarly, in the mutant Siamese cat exhibiting blindness in a visual hemifield, the brain might be judged to be normal unless specific techniques are applied to show the aberrant connections of subcortical and cortical visual structures (Guillery & Kass, 1971). In summary, therefore, the absence of demonstrated pathology cannot constitute evidence in favor of the contention that the brain is normal.

Except for the cases in the literature in which stuttering, aphasia, or a reading disorder in childhood can be readily traced to a specific acquired neurological event, the anatomy of specific language disorders in childhood is virtually unknown. In the acquired disorders, the brain pathology generally corresponds in location and histology to that found in adults with similar acquired disorders of language (Alajouanine & Lhermitte, 1965; Guttmann, 1942), albeit with some differences. For example, nonfluent aphasias in childhood can be seen with lesions located either posteriorly or anteriorly in the left cerebral hemisphere, whereas in the adult they are predominantly the consequence of anterior lesions (Benson & Geschwind, 1977). Most lesions, nevertheless, affect perisylvian (classical) language areas. In addition, deep lesions, especially in young children, appear to produce more long-lasting effects on language functions than similar unilateral lesions in the adult and older children (Dennis, personal communication). These observations suggest that even in the cases of acquired lesions resulting in language disturbances in childhood, the peculiarities of a developing nervous system must be considered more closely. Whether a lesion acquired early produces lesser (Kennard, 1940) or greater dysfunction (Schneider, 1979), it is clear that developmental issues having to do with postnatal brain growth come into play in acquired aphasias of children, but not in adults.

In the developmental disorders which are presumably not the result of an acquired lesion, the brain has by and large not been studied. There exist in the literature three exceptions: (1) a case of congenital aphasia with neuropathological findings (Landau, Goldstein, & Kleffner, 1960)[2]; (2) a case of developmental dyslexia with possible abnormalities in gross and microscopic cerebral morphology (Drake, 1968); and (3) a second case of developmental dyslexia with architectonic abnormalities in the cortex of the left hemisphere (Galaburda & Kemper, 1979) and in the posterior thalamus bilaterally (Galaburda & Eidelberg, 1982). In this chapter, the structural abnormalities in the last case will be reviewed in the light of knowledge of the normal anatomical organization of the brain for language function.

CASE REPORT[3]

The patient was born at term after a normal gestation and delivery. There were no neonatal complications and his early developmental milestones were judged to be normal. The only abnormality noted in early childhood was that the patient was clumsier than his siblings. Speech in full sentences was delayed until after the age of 3 years. Difficulties with reading and spelling were noted soon after entrance into elementary school, and he was made to repeat the first

---

[2]In this case, the nature of the lesion suggests that it was possibly acquired early in life.

[3]For a fuller account, the reader is referred to the original case description (Galaburda & Kemper, 1979).

grade. At that time, the diagnosis of specific developmental dyslexia was first made. A routine neurological evaluation disclosed no abnormal findings, and the Stanford-Binet intelligence score was 105. The patient's difficulties persisted despite special tutoring, and at 13 years he was given a battery of tests of intelligence and achievement with repeat testing at ages 14, 15, and 19 years. The test results showed that in spite of intelligence scores within or slightly below the average range, reading performance and spelling were well below expectation for his intellectual level, sociocultural opportunities, and educational exposure. Furthermore, although his arithmetical ability was thought to be better than his reading and writing, an evaluation done when the patient was 18 years of age placed this skill at the fourth-grade level. At the same time, mild difficulties with right–left orientation and finger recognition were noted. Tests of cerebral lateralization using dichotic digits showed a marked right-ear superiority, suggesting left-hemisphere control of language.

The patient developed nocturnal seizures at age 16 years that were easily controlled with phenytoin. At that time, repeated neurological examinations at a seizure clinic again failed to disclose any abnormalities except for the dyslexia. Routine electroencephalograms were normal except for one sleep study which showed borderline slowing over the right hemisphere. An isotope brain scan was normal.

The patient was left-handed, as were several other family members. He was the youngest of 4 siblings, 3 males and 1 female. Both brothers and the father (but not the sister or mother) were slow readers, albeit not to the degree exhibited by the patient. No other member of the family had seizures.

At age 18 years, the patient began training in sheet metal work. His work was deemed of excellent quality, and during his apprenticeship he was able to supplement his income by selling metal sculptures that he made. When he was 20 years old, 6 days after he began his first paying job, the patient died suddenly as the result of an accidental fall from a great height.

METHODS

The brain was embedded whole in celloidin and cut in gapless serial histological sections at a thickness of 35 μ. Every twentieth section was stained for myelin by the Loyez method, and the adjacent section with Nissl stain.

Analysis of the sections was carried out at the cytoarchitectonic and myeloarchitectonic level. Architectonics refers to the arrangement of cells, fibers, or other neural elements as seen under low-power magnification. Cortical cytoarchitectonics refers to the arrangement of neurons in the cortex into layers and columns and stresses additional features such as cell size and cell packing density. Myeloarchitectonics relies on the appearance of myelinated nerve fibers and their tangential and radial arrangements. Cytoarchitectonic analysis allows a given cellular structure (i.e., cortex or subcortical nucleus) to be regionally differentiated into separate areas. Distortions in architectonic appearance, especially if they are subtle, can easily escape standard neuropathological analysis of autopsied brains.

Findings in the Brain

Abnormalities in the Cortex

There were no gross abnormalities in the brain. Architectonic abnormalities were seen in the cortex of the left cerebral hemisphere and were of three types:

1. A large area of micropolygyria of the four-layered type was present in the posterior, superior temporal gyrus and obliterated almost completely the normal architecture of this region. Primarily affected by the malformation was architectonic area Tpt (discussed in what follows), but smaller portions of other auditory-related cortices were also involved.
2. Multiple areas of focal cortical dysplasia consisting of ectopic neurons were present in layer I and in the immediately subcortical white matter. These were found throughout the left hemisphere, but most densely in the posterior half, involving parietal, temporal, and occipital fields.
3. There were areas of disordered cortical architecture consisting of distortion of normal cortical layering and of the presence of abnormally large pyramidal neurons in the deeper layers, all considered to be primitive cortical features. These were seen in a distribution similar to that of the second type of abnormality, in addition to being found in the left cingulate gyrus.

Abnormalities of Subcortical White Matter

An abnormally increased width of the subcortical white matter was found in the left hemisphere. By comparison to age-matched controls, it appeared that the left white matter was too thick, rather than that the right was too narrow. Furthermore, the left hemisphere was wider than the right throughout its length, producing an abnormal pattern of hemispheric asymmetry. The uniform increase in left-sided white matter produced the appearance of a large left hemisphere.

Abnormalities in the Thalamus

The lateralis posterior and medial geniculate nuclei of the thalamus were abnormal bilaterally. In stained cell sections, the nuclei showed an excessive number of larger neurons which were abnormally placed dorsally in the nuclei. The myelin preparations showed even more clearly distortions in the shape of these nuclei as well as the presence of abnormal myelinated fiber tracts.

DISCUSSION

The interpretation of the findings in the dyslexic brain must be carried out in the light of the knowledge of the organization of the normal brain for language function. This knowledge has been obtained by the analysis of the effects on language and speech of localized lesions, occurring either naturally or as the result of surgery. Additional information on the localization of language in the brain has been gathered during brain stimulation at surgery and after electroencephalographic localization of epileptic phenomena altering language. Furthermore, the identification in animals, particularly in the nonhuman primates, of cortical regions homologous in architectonic structure to the human language areas has permitted the more detailed study of the cortico–cortical and cortico–subcortical connections which may also exist in the human brain to underlie language functions. Some of this knowledge is reviewed next.

Language Areas

On the basis of lesion data and electrophysiological experiments during neurosurgery, certain parts of the cortex and thalamus of the left hemisphere can be said to play a crucial role in language function. In the temporal lobe, an area of special importance is located in the caudal third of the superior temporal gyrus, a portion of the auditory representation in the cortex. Lesions in this area are apt to produce Wernicke's aphasia (Benson & Geschwind, 1977) and stimulation during surgery results in language disturbances (Whitaker & Ojemann, 1977). A gross anatomical landmark present in this region, the planum temporale, is significantly larger on the left side in about two-thirds of brains (Geschwind & Levitsky, 1968) and a cytoarchitectonic subdivision, area Tpt, tends to parallel this left–right asymmetry in favor of the left side (Galaburda, Sanides, & Geschwind, 1978). In man, the connections of this area are not specified other than by the general knowledge that a fiber bundle known as the arcuate fasciculus connects this region and the inferior parietal lobe to the inferior premotor and prefrontal areas in the frontal lobe. In rhesus monkey, a homologous cytoarchitectonic area on the posterior, superior temporal gyrus sends discrete projections to a specific area in the inferior premotor region (Pandya & Galaburda, 1980) as well as to the supplementary motor region (Pandya, Hallett, & Mukherjee, 1969), the inferior parietal lobule (Pandya & Seltzer, 1982), the posterior pericingulate area (Pandya & Seltzer, 1982), and the pulvinar-LP complex of the thalamus (Eidelberg & Galaburda, 1982). All of these connectionally related areas have been implicated in language control.

In the frontal lobe, another area of special interest is located in the posterior third of the inferior frontal gyrus. Lesions in this area may produce a Broca's aphasia (Benson & Geschwind, 1977), and language disturbances from stimulation in this area are also seen (Whitaker & Ojemann, 1977). The gross anatomy of this region is also asymmetrical in that more folding of cortex is seen on the left side (Eberstaller, 1884; Galaburda, 1980; Vignolo, personal communication). Present in this region, an architectonic area of distinct morphology by virtue of its pattern of lipofuscin accumulation was found to be significantly larger on the left in 6 out of 10 brains and larger on the right in 1 brain (Galaburda, 1980).

Additional areas are present in the inferior parietal lobule and in the medial hemisphere. Area 39 (of Brodmann) on the angular gyrus, when lesioned, can cause anomic aphasia as well as reading disturbances (Benson & Geschwind, 1977), and lesions in the midline of the hemisphere which damage the supplementary motor areas can result in transcortical aphasias (Ross, 1980; Rubens, 1975).

Both lesions and stimulation in the posterior left thalamus can produce transient aphasias of the anomic type as well as disturbances of speech output (Bell, 1968; Guiot, Hertzog, Rondot, & Molina, 1961; Ojemann, 1977). Judging from the location of the insult, the nuclear group most likely to be disrupted is the lateralis posterior–pulvinar complex. These thalamic nuclei, as surmised from comparative studies, are connected with the inferior premotor region, with area Tpt, and with the inferior parietal lobule (Eidelberg & Galaburda, 1982; Van Buren & Borke, 1972). Furthermore, asymmetries have been found in the LP nucleus, with 8 out of 9 brains showing a significant left-sided preponderance in volume (Eidelberg & Galaburda, 1982).

Gross Anatomical and Radiological Asymmetries

It is important to define gross anatomical asymmetries, and to relate these to laterality of behavioral measures, as such asymmetries are likely to be identified in living subjects, usually by the use of radiological techniques. The sylvian fissure is asymmetrical, especially in its posterior end, where it is shorter and curls upward on the right in the majority of right-handers (Hochberg & LeMay, 1975; LeMay & Culebras, 1972). Such an asymmetry may be partly the result of a large left temporal operculum. In fact, the excess in size of the left area Tpt may contribute to the sylvian asymmetry (Galaburda, Sanides, & Geschwind, 1978). Alternately, or in addition, the smaller, more vertical right fissure may reflect an underdevelopment of the right parietal operculum.

In CT scans, the right frontal lobe extends forward of the left and is wider. On the other hand, the left occipital lobe extends caudal to and is wider than the right (LeMay & Kido, 1978). A CT study on dyslexic patients showed that this pattern of petalia, as this phenomenon is termed, is more often reversed in dyslexics with speech delay and diminished verbal IQs (Hier, LeMay, Rosenberger, & Perlo, 1978). It is at least suggested by these studies that the anatomy of the brain in dyslexia may include abnormal manifestations of gross anatomical asymmetry and that these asymmetry variants may correlate with behavioral measures. The autopsy case reported here illustrated still another abnormal pattern of asymmetry, with wider entire left hemisphere.

The Dyslexic Brain

The dyslexic brain described in this chapter showed no gross abnormalities except for the unusual manifestation of asymmetry. Cursory examination of the external surface of the brain did not show evidence of acquired lesions or malformations. The sometimes described poverty of small sulci seen in mental retardation (Yakovlev, 1959) was not present. The micropolygyria escaped detection, as it often does until the brain is sectioned. On microscopic examination, there was remarkable cortical dysplasia with micropolygyria involving predominantly cytoarchitectonic area Tpt on the left planum temporale, and mild cortical dysplasias throughout the left hemisphere. The right cerebral cortex did not show anomalies.

The histological features of the micropolygyria conformed to those described in the literature for the four-layered type (Bielschowsky, 1920). Although the cause of this malformation is not known (Larroche, 1977), it is of interest to note that Bielschowsky (1920) considered that this type of cortex could result from the excessively slow migration of neuroblasts. The bizarreness of the cortical appearance has led others to invoke a more profound disorder of cortical formation, involving more than the migration period (Diezel, 1954).

In 6 of 16 cases reported by Brun (1975), there was a history suggestive of involvement by micropolygyric malformation in other members of the family. In 7 of these brains, the micropolygyria affected only small areas of the brain. It would be of great interest to see whether a familial form of micropolygyria localized to the perisylvain cortex on the left side could be responsible for the reading difficulties seen in some dyslexic patients and in their family members.

Thalamic abnormalities were found bilaterally in the reported case. The nature of these abnormalities is perplexing. However, relying on inquiries into the ontogenesis of the pulvinar—LP complex (Rakic, 1974), a model has been proposed to explain some elements of the pathology described here as well as the reported anatomical asymmetry in the normal posterior thalamus (Galaburda & Eidelberg, 1982). The ganglionic eminence is thought to serve as a "common fountainhead" for cells of telecephalic origin in the pulvinar—LP anlage, as well as the associated homotypical cortices. Based on this common origin, it is speculated that certain recognition properties are retained to allow for subsequent thalamocortical synapsis between these physically removed neuronal elements. In fact, ultrastructural studies in the pulvinar of the monkey have revealed the presence of unique synaptic relationships between the cortex and the pulvinar not demonstrable in the cortical projections to other thalamic nuclei. It is therefore plausible that a developmental interdependence exists between the pulvinar—LP complex and the associated areas of projection. It would thus be natural to expect corresponding asymmetries of the cortex and of a closely associated nuclear structure, both of which derive from a common pool of cells in which the propensity for asymmetry is perhaps genetically encoded. Furthermore, as the migrations of these parallel elements would be more or less concurrent, it might be reasonable to assume that a defect in the migration of cells to one element might likewise influence the migrational pattern of the other. Either a migrational (16–20 weeks) time scheme for the development of the micropolygyria or a postmigrational (20–27 weeks) scheme would be consistent with a concurrent developmental lesion in the posterior thalamus, as telecephalic cells migrate into the pulvinar–LP anlage wall through the end of the middle trimester, if not later. A postmigrational lesion is, however, less likely in light of the nature of the associated cortical lesions, particularly the focal disordering of cortical layering and the presence of ectopic neurons in the molecular layer of the auditory cortex. This view is also supported by the reported earlier cytoarchitectonic maturation of the posterior thalamus relative to the associated homotypical cortex in the early postmigrational period, rendering a secondary thalamic lesion less likely at that time. It seems, therefore, more reasonable to postulate that an aberration of migration gave rise to the micropolygyria as well as the other cortical dysplasias. The concurrently migrating cells destined for LP may have been similarly delayed in passage, thus giving rise to a late-arriving group positioned abnormally in that nucleus as described earlier. The dorsal position of the abnormal thalamic neurons is intriguing in light of Angevine's study of thalamic embryogenesis in the mouse in which later-generated cells tended to migrate dorsally (Angevine, 1970), although it is not clear that similar gradients apply in the migrations of the telencephalically derived cells of the human pulvinar–LP anlage.

Similarly, it is reasonable to postulate a developmental dependence between MGN and its target field (namely, layer 1 of the auditory cortices). The presence of cortical dysplasias in these areas might be reflected in similar distortions of the normal migrational pattern with a concomitant developmental disorganization in the MGN as described earlier. Indeed, it might be argued that the contralateral thalamic lesion described here arose by the same pathogenetic mechanism, that is, the same defect in neuronal migration extended to telencephalic cells which migrate along the midline. Although the existence of such a migration has not been demonstrated experimentally, autoradiographic demonstrations of bilaterality of connections from frontal association cortex to the dorsal thalamus in infant and juvenile monkeys make this a tenable hypothesis. If similar projections exist in the posterior association cortices, it might be advanced as an extension of the preceding arguments, that cells of telencephalic origin perhaps migrate across the midline (possibly through the corpus callosum which develops between the tenth and twentieth week) to populate the contralateral pulvinar–LP anlage. Common cellular recognition properties, as proposed earlier, would allow for the development of bilateral corticothalamic connections later on. Consequently, it is conceivable that a single defect in migration would give rise to bilateral thalamic lesions in the face of a unilateral cortical abnormality, as seen in the reported case.

Bilaterality of subcortical connections from the larger of two homologous asymmetrical cortical fields might reasonably be part of the substrate underlying cerebral dominance. Thus, it is quite possible that dominant cortical regions project more strongly bilaterally, as might be construed from studies that have shown that the right side of the spinal cord is likely to receive more pyramidal fibers than the left, evidently from the fact that the left pyramid tends to be more fully decussated than the right. A possible function for this type of asymmetry might thus be that the dominant hemisphere would have a bilateral outflow to subcortical structures and might, in fact, obstruct outflow from the minor side. In this scheme, only destruction of the dominant cortical area would release the opposite side, enabling it to express its previously suppressed function. It is therefore not surprising to encounter bilaterality of connections and of developmental lesions stemming from a developmental insult affecting a dominant cortical area in the case of dyslexia. As the thalamic receptor zones on both sides are abnormal, it seems reasonable that outflow from the intact hemisphere would be obstructed as well, leading to a permanent language disorder—dyslexia in this case. By analogy, if the dominant cortex were injured after birth, minor hemisphere outflow could still be expressed through normal subcortical channels with some recovery of function becoming possible.

The cause of the migrational abnormality in the dyslexic brain is not clear, although the possible heritable nature of the disorder in this case (see Galaburda & Kemper, 1979) might reflect a genetic defect in the cellular programming of neuronal migration as opposed to an extrinsic insult occurring at the time of migration.[4] The finding of cortical migration abnormalities in the cortex of only one side suggests the possibility that during development the left and right hemispheres (or specific regions within them) are partly under separate controls. Were these controls to produce asymmetries in rates of left and right cortical development, specific genetic lesions or pathological changes in the uterine environment might be expected to affect the hemispheres differentially during development. Thus, it is conceivable that a lesion in a gene will be reflected in pathology on one side and not the other. No such genetic lesion has been demonstrated in dyslexia, although the presence of the behavioral phenotype in familial dyslexia has been linked to the fifteenth chromosome (see Smith, Pennington, Kimberling, & Lubbs, Chapter 12, this volume). Likewise, acquired intrauterine insults might be felt more strongly on one side than the other, were the worse affected side to be at a more vulnerable developmental stage during the insult. In general, structures in a more primitive developmental stage are more likely to be injured. Thus, for instance, in congenital rubella, the clinical findings are more severe the earlier the infection (Cooper, et al. 1969). If the left hemisphere develops more slowly, it may thus be more vulnerable.

---

[4]It is not implied here that a specific gene codes for a specific program of neuronal migration and that a disruption in the genotype results in a disruption in the program. Rather, it is more likely that abnormal migration is the result of a "cascade of pleiotropic effects initiated by a [usually unknown] primary effect of a [genetic] mutation [p. 170]." (For an essay on the strengths and weaknesses of the genetic approach to neural development, see Stent, 1981.)

There is in fact evidence that, at the gross anatomical level, asymmetries in rates of hemispheral development exist (Chi, Dooling & Gilles, 1977; Fontes, 1944; Hervé, 1888). It seems that at least in perisylvian cortex, the appearance of secondary and tertiary sulci occurs first on the right side (see Figure 5.1). It is not possible to state with certainty the stage of development at which the right side accelerates ahead of the left. The possibilities include an asymmetry in the rate of development of the neuropil at the cortical site, the increased rates of right-sided development beginning at earlier stages (e.g., DNA replication, mitosis, or cell migration), or an asymmetry in the rates of cell death during the final stages of cortical modeling. The identification of animal models showing similar developmental asymmetries will be needed to further pinpoint the mechanisms behind the development of these asymmetries as well as the biological parameters that could alter this asymmetrical development. The findings in the dyslexic brain, which essentially point to a form of unilateral developmental arrest, may represent an extreme manifestation of the normally occurring asymmetry in development of the cortex of the two hemispheres. Unlike the situation in the normal, however, the developing left hemisphere of the dyslexic may run out of time, and thus be unable to conclude its normal development.

Finally, it is interesting to note that the dichotic listening test was lateralized to the left hemisphere in the reported dyslexic patient. This finding is consistent with certain data pointing out that strong lateralization of language to the left hemisphere may not be compatible with the highest level of performance. Thus females, who generally perform better in verbal tests than males, appear to be less lateralized as tested by dichotic syllables (Lake & Bryden, 1976; Springer & Searleman, 1978). A corollary to this is the finding that the 45 (XO) phenotypic females who perform much better in verbal than visual tests are less lateralized for verbal function to the left hemisphere (see Nettley, Chapter 13, this volume). Conversely, males and androgenized females with relatively poorer verbal performance are more lateralized to the left hemisphere for language function. One could construct a model in which a slowly developing left hemisphere allows invasion of the left by right hemisphere skills, thus leading to a restricted and highly lateralized language function in the left hemisphere. Conversely, a faster developing left hemisphere would itself be capable of invading the right side, thus producing expansion and bilateralization of language representation in that brain. The existence of such physiological "invasion" of an inhibited hemisphere by its uninhibited mate is suggested by the experiment of Cynader, Leporé, and Guillemot (1981), in which a hemisphere artificially rendered visually handicapped during development is functionally invaded by the other. At the anatomical level, cell death and rerouting of axons may occur during development in the presence of early lesions (Goldman, 1979; Innocenti, 1981; Schneider, 1970), thus providing anatomical substrates for dramatic functional reorganization. Such rerouting, if directed toward the left hemisphere, might explain the presence of excessive white matter on the left, thus resulting in the type of asymmetry shown by the brain of the dyslexic patient.

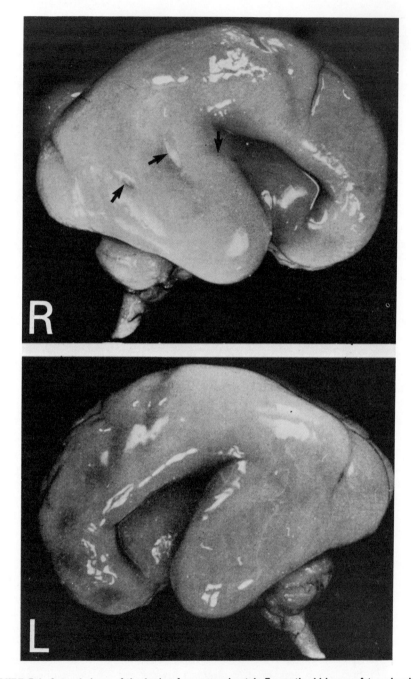

FIGURE 5.1. Lateral views of the brain of an approximately 5-month-old human fetus showing the asymmetry in sulcation of perisylvian temporal cortex. Note the presence of sulci on the right (top, arrows).

REFERENCES

Alajouanine, T., & Lhermitte, F. Acquired aphasia in children. *Brain*, 1965, *88*, 653–662.

Angevine, J. B., Jr. Time of neuron origin in the diencephalon of the mouse: An autoradiographic study. *Journal of Comparative Neurology*, 1970, *139*, 177–188.

Bell, D. S. Speech functions of the thalamus inferred from the effects of thalamotomy. *Brain*, 1968, *91*, 619–638.

Benson, D. F., & Geschwind, N. The aphasias and related disturbances. In A. B. Baker & L. H. Baker (Eds.), *Clinical neurology* (Vol. 1). Hagerstown, Md.: Harper & Row, 1977.

Bielschowsky, M. Zur Histopathologie und Pathogenese der amaurotischen Idiotic mit besonderer Berücksichtigung der Zerebellaren Veränderungen. *Journal für Psychologie und Neurologie* (Leipzig), 1920, *26*, 123–199.

Brun, A. The subpial granular layer of the foetal cerebral cortex in man. *Acta Pathol. Microbiol. Scand.* [Suppl.], 1975, *179*, 40.

Chi, J. G., Dooling, E. C., & Gilles, F. H. Gyral development of the human brain. *Annals of Neurology*, 1977, *1*, 86–93.

Clairborne, J. H. Types of congenital symbol amblyopia. *Journal of the American Medical Association*, 1906, *47*, 1813–1816.

Cooper, L. Z., Ziring, P. R., Ockerse, A. B., Fedun, B. A., Kelly, B., & Krujman, S. Rubella: Clinical manifestations and management. *American Journal of Disease of Children*, 1969, *118*, 18–29.

Critchley, M. *Developmental dyslexia*. London: William Heinemann, 1964.

Cynader, M., Leporé, F., & Guillemot, J.-P. Inter-hemispheric competition during post natal development. *Nature*, 1981, *290*, 139–140.

Diezel, P. B. Microgyrie infolge cerebraler Speicheldrüsen—Virusinfektion im Rahmen einer generalisierten Cytomegalie bei einem Säugling. *Virchows Archiv*, 1954, *325*, 109–130.

Drake, W. E. Clinical and pathological findings in a child with a developmental learning disability. *Journal of Learning Disabilities*, 1968, *1*, 9–25.

Eberstaller, O. Zur Oberflächenanatomie der Grosshorn Hemisphären. *Wiener Medizinische Blätter*, 1884, *7*, pp. 479, 642, 644.

Eidelberg, D., & Galaburda, A. M. Symmetry and asymmetry in the human posterior thalamus, I: Cytoarchitectonic analysis in normals. *Archives of Neurology*, 1982, *39*, 325–332.

Fontes, V. *Mortologia do córtex cerebral*. Lisboa: Instituto de Antonia Aurelio da Costa Ferreira, 1944.

Galaburda, A. M. La région de Broca: Observations anatomiques faites un siècle après la mort de son découvreur. *Revue Neurologique*, 1980, *136*, 609–616.

Galaburda, A. M., & Eidelberg, D. Symmetry and asymmetry in the human posterior thalamus, II: Thalamic lesions in a case of developmental dyslexia. *Archives of Neurology*, 1982, *39*, 333–336.

Galaburda, A. M., & Kemper, T. Cytoarchitectonic abnormalities in developmental dyslexia: A case study. *Annals of Neurology*, 1979, *6*, 94–100.

Galaburda, A. M., Sanides, F., & Geschwind, N. Human brain: Cytoarchitectonic left–right asymmetries in the temporal speech region. *Archives of Neurology*, 1978, *35*, 812–817.

Geschwind, N., & Levitsky, W. Human brain: Left–right asymmetries in temporal speech region. *Science*, 1968, *161*, 186–189.

Goldman, P. S. Contralateral projections to the dorsal thalamus from frontal association cortex in the rhesus monkey. *Brain Research*, 1979, *166*, 166–171.

Guillery, R. W., & Kaas, J. H. A study of normal and congenitally abnormal retinogeniculate projections in cats. *Journal of Comparative Neurology*, 1971, *143*, 73–100.

Guiot, G., Hertzog, E., Rondot, P., & Molina, P. Arrest or acceleration of speech evoked by thalamic stimulation in the course of stereotaxic procedures for Parkinsonism. *Brain*, 1961, *84*, 363–379.

Guttman, E. Aphasia in children. *Brain*, 1942, *65*, 205–219.

Hervé, G. *La circonvolution de Broca*. Paris: Delahaye & Lecrosnier, 1888.

Hier, D. B., LeMay, M., Rosenberger, P. B., & Perlo, V. Developmental dyslexia. *Archives of Neurology*, 1978, *35*, 90–92.

Hinshelwood, J. *Congenital word-blindness*. London: Lewis, 1917.

Hochberg, F. H., & LeMay, M. Arteriographic correlates of handedness. *Neurology*, 1975, *25*, 48–222.

Innocenti, G. M. Growth and reshaping of axons in the establishment of visual callosal connections. *Science*, 1981, *212*, 824–826.

Kennard, M. A. Relation of age to motor impairment in man and in subhuman primates. *Archives of Neurology and Psychiatry*, 1940, *44*, 377–397.

Lake, D., & Bryden, M. Handedness and sex differences in hemispheric asymmetry. *Brain and Language*, 1976, *3*, 266–282.

Landau, W. M., Goldstein, R., & Kleffner, F. R. Congenital aphasia: A clinicopathologic study. *Neurology*, 1960, *10*, 915–921.

Larroche, J. C. Cytoarchitectonic abnormalities (abnormalities of cell migration). In P. J. Vinken & G. W. Bruyn (Eds.), *Handbook of clinical neurology*. Amsterdam: North-Holland, 1977.

LeMay, M., & Culebras, A. Human brain: Morphologic differences in the hemisphere demonstrated by carotid arteriography. *New England Journal of Medicine*, 1972, *287*, 168–170.

LeMay, M., & Kido, D. K.: Asymmetries of the cerebral hemispheres on computed tomograms. *J. Comp. Assist. Tomogr.*, 1978, *2*, 471–476.

Ojemann, G. S. Asymmetric function of the thalamus in man. *Annals of the New York Academy of Sciences*, 1977, *299*, 380–396.

Pandya, D. N., & Galaburda, A. M. Role of architectonics and connections in the study of primate brain evolution. *American Journal of Physical Anthropology*, 1980, *52*, 197.

Pandya, D. N., Hallett, M., & Mukherjee, S. K. Intra- and interhemispheric connections of the neocortical auditory system in rhesus monkeys. *Brain Research*, 1969, *14*, 49–65.

Pandya, D. N., & Seltzer, B. Intrinsic connections and architectonics of the posterior parietal cortex in the rhesus monkey. *Journal of Comparative Neurology*, 1982, *204*, 196–210.

Rakic, P. The embryonic development of the pulvinar–LP complex in man. In I. S. Cooper, M. Risklan, & P. Rakic (Eds.), *The pulvinar–LP complex*. Springfield, Ill.: Charles C Thomas, 1974.

Ross, E. Left medial parietal lobe and receptive language functions: Mixed transcortical aphasia after left anterior cerebral artery infarction. *Neurology*, 1980, *30*, 144–151.

Rubens, A. B. Aphasia with infarction in the territory of the anterior cerebral artery. *Cortex*, 1975, *11*, 239–250.

Schneider, G. E. Mechanisms of functional recovery following lesions of visual cortex or superior colliculus in neonate and adult hamsters. *Brain, Behavior, and Evolution*, 1970, *3*, 295–323.

Schneider, G. E. Is it really better to have your brain lesion early? A revision of the "Kennard Principle." *Neuropsychologia*, 1979, *17*, 557–583.

Springer, S., & Searleman, A. The ontogeny of hemispheric specialization: Evidence from dichotic listening in twins. *Neuropsychologia*, 1978, *16*, 269–281.

Stent, G. S. Strength and weakness of the genetic approach to the development of the nervous system. *Annual Review of Neuroscience*, 1981, *4*, 163–194.

Van Buren, J., & Borke, R. *Variations and connections of the human thalamus* (Vols. 1 & 2). New York: Springer, 1972.

Whitaker, H. A., & Ojemann, G. A. Graded localization of learning from electrical stimulation of left cerebral cortex. *Nature*, 1977, *270*, 50–51.

Yakovlev, P. I. Anatomy of the human brain and the problem of mental retardation. In P. W. Bowman & H. V. Mantner (Eds.), *Mental retardation: Proceedings of the First International Conference on Mental Retardation*. New York: Grune & Stratton, 1959.

6

Sex Differences: Clues or Myths on Genetic Aspects of Speech and Language Disorders?[1]

PAUL SATZ
JOSEF ZAIDE

The present chapter falls within the section on definition of phenotype and is concerned with anatomical, physiological, and behavioral attributes of speech and language disorders. Definition of *phenotype* is obviously a first step in any attempt to identify those factors intrinsically or extrinsically related to the phenotype. Here we shall focus on the problem of *sex* differences and examine whether this variable deserves special treatment in the investigation of biological mechanisms on various behavioral attributes of speech and language disorders in children. Before beginning this discussion, it might be helpful to review some definitional issues concerning terms such as *phenotype* and *sex* in genetic research.

Wittig (1979) provides a useful statement on the concept of inheritance as it relates to phenotype.

> It is clear that *what one inherits* are the genes (or, more specifically, the amino acid sequences of protein they represent). Taken together, these inherited entities constitute one's *genotype*. The fundamental problem with which the genetic analysis of the development of human behavior is concerned is understanding the ways in which one's genotype expresses itself. The individual's *phenotype* is the set of observable outcomes resulting from the integration of genetic and developmental experiences (Tobach, 1972). Because the genotype is not directly observable, the phenotype is the datum that developmentalists must work with, regardless of the purpose of the investigation, the methods employed, the comparisons to be made, or the uses to which the information is ultimately put. Because the phenotype is really conditioned by the interplay of genes and environment, Dobzhansky (1973)

[1]This research was supported in part by funds from an NIH grant (7 ROI NS 18462–01) entitled *Laterality of Sensory and Motor Functions in Man.*

GENETIC ASPECTS OF
SPEECH AND LANGUAGE DISORDERS

employs the term "genetic conditioning" in order to emphasize the fact that heredity is a process rather than a permanent state. Use of the term "environmental conditioning" would be equally correct, emphasizing the fact that the degree to which a given genotype is expressed in a particular phenotype is dependent on the environmental conditions to which it is exposed. In contrast, what is *genetically determined*, in Dobzhansky's (1973) view, is the range of reactions obtainable under all possible environmental conditions (i.e., the range of potential phenotypes). However, the phenotype actually expressed is restricted by the particular set of environments to which the genes are exposed [p. 24].

Another confusion in developmental research concerns the manner in which the term *sex* is defined. Wittig (1979) is instructive on this issue as well.

Age, like sex, can function as a stimulus variable as well as a subject variable. As subject variables, age and sex cannot be randomly assigned and their use as independent variables in experimental studies does not justify concluding that variation in behavior associated with such factors has been caused by them. Such variables may also function as a stimulus to others, whose behavior may well be changed owing to the sex or age of the person with whom they are interacting. Because it is possible, in an experiment, to randomly assign individuals to interact with one or another stimulus person and the age or sex of these stimulus persons may be varied systematically, the use of such variables does allow one to draw cause–effect inferences. When using sex or age as stimulus variables, however, it is necessary to keep in mind that the stimulus person's age or sex may be contributing to the reaction merely because of an age or sex bias on the part of the respondent, rather than because of any quality inherent in the ages or sexes under study [p. 23].

Morgan (1980) raises a similar concern with respect to how the term sex is defined in the investigation of differences on an attribute or trait. To conclude that a difference on a phenotype is more marked in men than in women

anticipates an ambiguity that is still found in the literature on "sex differences." Is the trait supposed to be sexually dimorphic, as the language above suggests, or does it imply that sex had some influence on observed variation in the character? The distinction is an important one. Sexual dimorphism refers to a state of affairs in which individual members of the two sexes can be distinguished by one or more features, such as the secondary sexual characteristics. On the other hand, there are traits such as height, in terms of which large populations of the two sexes may differ on average, but which would be quite useless for determining whether an individual were male or female. The term "sex difference" can refer to either of those states of affairs, and one could therefore argue that it is not sufficiently precise for scientific usage. Could not much misunderstanding be avoided if we adopted a more refined terminology? I tentatively suggest that it might be useful to speak of sexual dimorphism when this is meant, and in other cases to speak of the influence of sex upon variation of the trait in question [pp. 244–245.].

The preceding comments, although familiar to behavioral geneticists, may not be so to neuropsychologists who have recently been attracted to the search for sex differences in cerebral lateralization. These comments address defini-

tional issues that must be confronted before any attempts at hypothesis generation or hypothesis testing are made.

With the preceding as background, it might be well to begin this discussion
by addressing the question of why sex differences should be examined at all in
the study of genetic aspects of speech and language disorders. Unfortunately, it
is difficult to justify why sex differences should be examined. At present, we lack
a firm data base as well as a conceptual framework for prosecuting such
research. On the other hand, the general topic of *sex differences* has in recent
years attracted considerable attention in the psychological literature. This literature, for the sake of convenience, can be divided into three areas: (*a*) *cognitive*
abilities, (*b*) *cerebral lateralization,* and (*c*) *prevalence attack rates* in speech-
and language-disabled children. The first two areas have largely been concerned with studies of normal non-brain-injured subjects.

SEX DIFFERENCES IN COGNITIVE ABILITIES

Demonstration of reliable sex differences in information-processing abilities would provide a logical first step in the process of seeking answers to these
putative differences. If it could be established that such differences exist on an
attribute, then studies could be launched to identify the mechanisms, intrinsic
and/or extrinsic, that might account for these differences. Following Maccoby
and Jacklin's classic review, *The Psychology of Sex Differences* (1974), claims
were made that differences had been established in three domains of intellectual functioning: mathematics, spatial visualization, and language processing.
Briefly, it was concluded that *in adolescence* sex differences emerged favoring
males in mathematical ability and spatial visualization (e.g., mental rotations)
and females in language-processing ability. These claims, largely premature,
soon triggered the interest of neuropsychologists and neurologists who had
long noted the association between these cognitive attributes and their hemispheric substrates. Even more striking was the presumption that these cognitive
abilities were compromised in children with speech and language disorders.
Hence, the stage was set: (1) males and females possess different cognitive–intellectual structures which (2) are known to be mediated differentially by
the two cerebral hemispheres; consequently, (3) there must be intrinsic sex
differences in the cerebral organization of these functional attributes.

But what is the evidence for the first postulate—namely, that there are sex
differences in cognitive ability? The evidence, unfortunately, is weak. Because
most of the literature is summarized in Maccoby and Maccoby and Jacklin
(1974), it might be instructive to quote from Fairweather's (1976) insightful,
though seldom quoted, review of that volume.

> Good and bad studies alike get equal weight; one positive finding gets (at least in
> the "difference" column) as much mention as numerous negative results in the

same or follow-up studies; table headings themselves may denote "parcel" areas without in reality admitting of the corresponding "parcel" answers they tempt; some areas (reading is a notable example) may fall in the gaps between tables; and finally, even allowing the accuracy, such a numerous "no difference" is a difficult story to remember, and may in turn obscure the few clear findings. Methodological problems are also given short shrift. Tendencies to use simplest of statistics, or none at all; to argue from single-sex studies; for one well-published positive finding to be remembered where a score of subsequent failures-to-replicate are forgotten; and the retreat-to-neutrality inherent in standardizations of many widely-used test batteries (omission of items yielding large sex-differences); all these alluded to, but rarely dealt with in depth. One looks in vain for a solid discussion of sex-of-experimentor effects. One final, perhaps forgivable affliction is that curious North American disease "Myopia USA." Much of the European, and notably British literature is missing, regrettably so, since such studies have been much less prone to spectacular findings, especially in childhood [pp. 233–234].

Fairweather's commentary should caution any premature pronouncements of "established" sex differencies in cognitive function. The weight of the evidence for such putative difference is weak, particularly for *verbal* abilities. Sex-related differences in *spatial* ability, although more often reported, are nevertheless subject to similar criticisms. The main issue concerns the problem of reliability. With respect to spatial abilities, Maccoby and Jacklin (1974) found such differences in only about 60% of the studies reviewed. Although these differences, unlike those of verbal abilities, have almost always been in the direction of higher male performance, the overlap between groups has been striking. In fact, Petersen (1981) has noted that "the variability *among* females and *among* males is always larger than the variability between males and females [p. 44]." Also, most studies in which differences have been reported have failed to correct for unequal variances between groups which would render the results invalid. Finally, where differences on a trait (verbal or spatial) have been demonstrated, the magnitude of these differences has been small, especially in terms of the proportion of variance accounted for by the attribute (Kinsbourne, 1980). Given this state of affairs, Jacklin (1979) has concluded that "looking for mechanisms to explain trivially small differences may be an exercise in futility [p. 368]." Fairweather (1976), in a similar vein, surmised that "what had before been a possibility at best slenderly evidenced, was widely taken for fact; and 'fact' hardened into 'biological dogma' [p. 233]."

The search for biological mechanisms presumed to underlie these sex differences in cognitive abilities, even though "slenderly evidenced," also failed to consider equally plausible alternative explanations—namely, sex-role socialization effects. This neglect is evident in the anthology edited by Wittig and Petersen, *Sex-Related Differences in Cognitive Functioning* (1979), only two chapters of which are devoted to socialization factors. The evidence reviewed in these two chapters provides compelling arguments for the role of masculine identification and social reinforcement factors in mathematical and spatial visualization performance. More importantly, these studies have shown that factors in the social milieu (home and school), which may have selectively biased earlier studies, may now be changing—including sex-related differences. These changes may encompass verbal abilities as well as spatial ones. In the 1973 national sample of high-school students taking college entrance tests, no sex-related differences in verbal abilities were found (Jacklin, 1979).

A further problem is that results showing sex differences in cognitive function could also have been biased by subject selection problems. In a multi-faceted study of spatial performance in males and females, Petersen (1981) has found that follow-up results were biased by a large dropout rate of males in the low-spatial-ability range. This finding suggests that volunteer samples may produce inherent selection biases in such studies.

Another compelling alternative explanation for sex differences in cognitive function relates to Waber's concept of maturation rate. She postulated that variation in maturational rate probably reflects endocrinological differences that affect both growth and cognitive processes. Since, according to Waber (1977), "the initiation of the hormonal events preceding puberty and the attainment of 'peak height velocity' (the point of most rapid acceleration in growth and height) occur earlier in females than in males, females may be considered to the early-maturing individuals in comparison to males. This difference in growth rates (and implicit endrocrinological correlates) may be related to reported differences in cognitive function [p. 29]." Implicit to this position, of course, is the assumption of marked individual differences within males and females in the rate of physical maturation. Waber (1977) advanced two hypotheses that purport to account for most of the interindividual variation on verbal and spatial tasks. Hypothesis I stated that early-maturing adolescents perform better than late-maturing adolescents on verbal tasks, and late-maturing adolescents perform better than early maturers on spatial tasks. Hypothesis II stated that early maturers perform better on verbal than on spatial tasks and that late maturers perform better on spatial than on verbal tasks. The critical test is Hypothesis I which involves a between-individuals comparison. Results partially confirmed this hypothesis; late-maturing adolescents, who were classified by Tanner's staging criteria for secondary sexual development (Marshall & Tanner, 1970), performed better than early maturers on a variety of spatial tasks. No between-individual effect, however, was observed for the verbal tasks. Hypothesis II was fully confirmed and showed that, independent of sex, early maturers performed better on verbal tasks and late maturers on spatial tasks. In other words, these results demonstrated that maturation rate, rather than sex, accounted for most of the variation on these cognitive traits.

The preceding comments have been made largely to dispel those pronouncements that continue to claim spectacular findings concerning sex-related differences in cognitive abilities. Although such differences may exist, at least for some cognitive attributes whose construct validity is still unspecified, the differences are hardly robust and may, in fact, be evanescent. These comments should therefore caution attempts to uncover causes for differences in an attribute that may not be real. Such skepticism was evident some 70 years ago in the writings of Helen Thompson Wooley on the topic of sex-related differences in cognitive ability (quoted in Parlee, 1978): "There is perhaps no field aspiring to be scientific where flagrant personal bias, logic martyred in the cause of supporting a prejudice, unfounded assertions, and even sentimental rot and drivel, have run riot to such an extent as here [p. 62]."

SEX DIFFERENCES IN CEREBRAL LATERALIZATION

Despite the problems of whether a sex-related difference in cognitive ability exists, neuropsychologists proceeded with vigor to ascertain the neural substrate for these presumed cognitive differences. The answer was soon forthcoming in the form of "cerebral dominance," although the logic for this formulation still remains obscure. On the basis of a few empirical studies employing normal subjects (perceptual asymmetries) and brain-injured patients (psychometric asymmetries), it was concluded that females are *less lateralized* than males in terms of language and visuospatial function in the brain. This spectacular claim, based on somewhat tenuous data and on no clear logical or theoretical framework, also implied that these phenotypic differences in hemispheric organization were sexually dimorphic; that is, that the brains of females are intrinsically different from the brains of males (McGlone, 1980). Such speculation calls to mind Fairweather's (1976) statement that "a possibility at best slenderly evidenced, was widely taken for fact; and 'fact' hardened into 'biological dogma' [p. 233]."

The position that females are less lateralized than males, extensively treated in a review by McGlone (1980), can be faulted on both conceptual and methodological grounds.

Conceptual Problems

A first conceptually based concern relates to the presumption that, by adolescence, language abilities are more highly developed in females and that spatial visualization abilities are more highly developed in males. If so, how can it be that females are less completely lateralized for both functions in which they excell (i.e., verbal) and functions in which they lag (i.e., spatial visualization) while males are more completely lateralized for functions in which they lag (i.e., verbal) and excell (i.e., spatial visualization)? The logic is obscure. In fact, the reasoning is so loose that it has led some investigators to quite the opposite claims. For example, Buffery and Gray (1972) conclude, on equally obscure grounds, that the male advantage in spatial visualization abilities is due to their bilateral (i.e., less completely lateralized) representation of spatial skills in the brain. A counsel of despair, indeed. Without a unifying theoretical framework, one is unable to *predict* whether the type of cerebral organization (unilateral or bilateral) would confer an advantage or disadvantage in terms of information-processing functions. As such, the conceptual link between the type of cerebral organization and speech and language disorders cannot be made.[2]

A second concern relates to the claim, often made, that these phenotypic sex–brain differences are not apparent until adolescence—at which time, incidentally, sex-role socialization factors have their maximum effects on behavior (Nash, 1979; Fox, Tobin, & Brady, 1979). If these phenotypic differences are not present during childhood, as even McGlone (1980) admits, then how are the presumed differences in cerebral specialization to be explained at adolescence? The logic is obscure. Note that this position rests on only marginal evidence of a sex-related difference in verbal ability at adolescence and even less evidence during childhood. On this most tenuous basis, McGlone (1980) then postulates a neural substrate which is presumed to be sexually dimorphic—that is, unilateral representation of speech in males and bilateral representation of speech in females—but only at adolescence! Notwithstanding such speculation, how does she account for the *change* in cerebral specialization within sexes over time? The answer is not at all clear.

Waber (1977) attempted to resolve this dilemma by invoking a lag mechanism which is presumed to delay physical and cognitive maturation, leading, by adolescence, to greater cerebral specialization of speech in later maturers, most of whom are boys. Only marginal support for this hypothesis was reported by Waber (1977) with negative results being reported by Petersen (1979). More recently, Waber (1979) revised this position by claiming that early maturers, most of whom are females, show more rapid acquisition of speech and language functions during childhood which is associated with greater cerebral lateralization during this developmental period. By adolescence, the language advantage in females attenuates, perhaps due to a ceiling effect, which results in a less complete form of hemispheric speech organization in early maturing females. Waber (1979) states that "despite the fact that females appear to be more lateralized in childhood, males are more lateralized as adults [p. 182]." This position can be critized on the following grounds:

1. It presumes a female advantage in verbal cognitive tasks during childhood rather than at adolescence, which is discrepant with most of the literature already reviewed.

2. It states that this cognitive advantage has an underlying neural substrate

---

[2]It has been suggested that an atypical form of cerebral speech dominance may underlie some types of dyslexia (Witelson, 1976; Zurif & Carson, 1970). This hypothesis likewise suffers on conceptual grounds because it postulates a form of incomplete hemispheric specialization that McGlone (1980) proposes for normal females, the vast majority of whom are known to be at low risk for dyslexia. Empirically, the hypothesis has also failed to receive any firm support in the literature (Satz, 1976). One might ask, however, whether McGlone's (1980) sexual dimorphism position would have any relevance for understanding some of the speech and language disorders. As it is presently formulated, approximately half of the normal adult population (i.e., females) are predicted to have an atypical form of hemispheric specialization. This position permits few degrees of freedom for addressing hemispheric substrates in abnormal development.

during childhood—namely, greater cerebral lateralization of speech in early maturers, most of whom are females. There is not one shred of evidence to support this claim and considerable evidence to disclaim it (Kinsbourne, 1980; McGlone, 1980; Bryden, 1981).

3. It postulates a developmental reversal in the cerebral lateralization of speech in both early and late maturers, which is not only absurd but also discrepant with current knowledge concerning the developmental invariance of speech lateralization in children and adults (Kinsbourne & Hiscock, 1977; Woods & Teuber, 1977; Satz & Bullard-Bates, 1981).

The preceding comments highlight some of the conceptual problems that afflict the proponents of the sex–brain dimorphism position. The following section examines briefly some of the methodological problems. What is the evidence upon which this intriguing though conceptually loose construct rests?

Methodological Problems

Claims that the brains of females are less functionally lateralized than those of males rest on two different methods of study. The first approach is based on studies of cognitive function (primarily WAIS Verbal and Performance IQ comparisons) in unilaterally brain-injured adults. The second approach is based on studies of perceptual asymmetries (dichotic listening and visual half-field recognition tasks) in non-brain-injured college students.

Clinical Studies

According to McGlone (1980), the major support for the position that there are sex differences in lateralization rests on studies of unilaterally brain-injured adults. In the introduction to her 1976 monograph, McGlone had stated regarding such studies that "findings, however, have been transitory (Lansdell, 1962), unreplicable (Lansdell & Urbach, 1965; Lansdell, 1968) or suggestive but not statistically significant (McGlone & Kertesz, 1973). Accordingly, McGlone (1976) undertook more systematic re-examination of the problem. She reported the following results:

1. The incidence of aphasia, following left-hemisphere damage was three times higher in the males than in the females.
2. The degree of aphasia was more severe in the males.
3. Verbal IQ scores were significantly lower than performance IQ scores in only the male sample following left-hemisphere damage.
4. Verbal memory performance (immediate and delayed) was also lower in only the male sample following left-hemisphere damage.

On the basis of these results she concluded that language functions were bilaterally represented in the female brain.

There are a number of flaws in this study that deserve mention. First, despite the higher incidence of aphasia in males, none of these patients came from the right-hemisphere-damaged group. A hypothesis of bilateral representation of speech in females would predict a higher proportion of crossed aphasias in females following right-sided damage. Second, the lower incidence of aphasia in females, following left-sided damage, directly contradicts her interpretation of bilateral speech representation in these patients. It has been shown that the incidence of aphasia following unilateral injury increases dramatically in cases of known or suspected bilateral speech representation (Satz, 1979; 1980; Carter, Hohenegger, and Satz, 1980). Third, the higher incidence of aphasia in her male sample may have been an artifact of lesion bias. It is well known that vascular injuries to the brain are more frequent in males than in females (Kertesz, 1981; Kinsbourne, 1980); McGlone's left-damaged male sample had proportionately more vascular as opposed to tumor etiologies. The slower onset of tumor damage permits more compensation by the intact brain (Kinsbourne, 1980). Kinsbourne (1980) has also noted that within McGlone's tumor group the left-damaged females had a higher proportion of less severe extrinsic tumors (meningiomas) as compared to intrinsic ones (gliomas). Fourth, McGlone's statement that the degree of aphasia was more severe in males is incorrect; the interaction between sex and degree of aphasia was not significant. Fifth, the interaction between sex and lesion side on Verbal IQ and verbal memory was weakened by the absence of a non-brain-injured control group in these comparisons. Also, these results could also have been biased by known differences in etiology and lesion severity between males and females.

In a follow-up study, McGlone (1978) reported somewhat similar results on the Verbal and Performance Scales of the WAIS. Right-handed males showed Verbal IQ deficits following left-hemisphere lesions and Performance IQ deficits following right-hemisphere lesions whereas right-handed females failed to show selective verbal or performance intellectual deficits after unilateral injury. Closer inspection of this study, however, suggests that the brain-injured sample was essentially the same as that used in the earlier study (1976). In fact, the sample sizes and lesion by sex distributions were almost identical in the two studies (Study 1: 32 male and 20 female left-sided lesions, 23 male and 17 female right-sided lesions; Study 2: 23 male and 20 female left-sided lesions, 17 male and 17 female right-sided lesions). It should be noted, however, that in the earlier study McGlone was unable to find a Performance IQ decline in either sex group following right-sided damage. Hence, one must ask whether the double dissociation reported in the 1978 study was due to *removal* of 9 males from the left-hemisphere group and 6 males from the right-hemisphere group in the earlier study (1976). The distribution of females by lesion side was identical in both studies.

Regardless of whether the study sample was essentially the same in both studies, the results are again open to criticism because of the failure to use a normal non-brain-injured comparison group in the determination of the respective Verbal and Performance IQ "deficits." It has long been known that sizable discrepancies between Verbal and Performance IQ can occur in the normal population (Matarazzo, 1972). Hence, without a standardization comparison, how could one interpret a discrepancy score, let alone a deficit score?

In defense of McGlone's (1980) sexual dimorphism position, Inglis and Lawson (1981) reviewed much of the literature on Verbal and Performance IQ discrepancies in unilaterally brain-injured adults. Although sex was seldom treated as a subject variable in these studies, they reasoned that this factor may have accounted for the failure to find a consistent test-specific laterality effect on the WAIS (only 5 of 14 studies reported positive findings). Inglis and Lawson (1981) further reasoned that if McGlone's (1980) position were valid, one would expect to find a higher proportion of males in the positive studies ($N = 5$) and, conversely, a lower proportion of males in the negative studies ($N = 9$). Although such a trend was found, the proportions were not significantly different. Yet the authors claimed the trend supported McGlone's (1980) position. They also reanalyzed the data from one of the nine studies that had reported negative results (Meyer & Jones, 1957), and found the test-specific laterality effect in the males ($N = 16$) but not in the females ($N = 15$). On the basis of this reanalysis, and the trend regarding proportion of males in the studies, the authors then extrapolated to the other eight negative studies and concluded that McGlone's position was unequivocally supported. This extrapolation is both unwarranted and extremely speculative. Their results merely narrow the rather wide discrepancy between positive and negative studies by one (six positive versus eight negative), leaving the role of sex effects unknown.

The major test of the bilaterality hypothesis in females would be in aphasia research. This approach circumvents many of the measurement and design problems inherent in psychometric studies such as the WAIS. If valid, one should expect to see a higher overall incidence of aphasia in females regardless of lesion side and a higher incidence of crossed aphasia or alexia following right-sided damage. There is not one shred of evidence to date, even in McGlone's (1976) study, to support this prediction. In fact, her results were contrary to the hypothesis. Moreover, two carefully controlled studies (Kertesz & Sheppard, 1981; Kertesz, 1981) subsequently failed to reveal a sex difference in the incidence or severity of aphasia or acquired alexia following unilateral brain injury. Nor did these studies find any evidence of crossed aphasia in females. It should be noted that these studies are strengthened by their quantitative assessment of aphasia and alexia and by their control for higher stroke incidence in males.

Studies with Normals

The search for sex differences in hemispheric speech lateralization in normal subjects has been conducted using primarily auditory verbal or visual verbal laterality procedures. Critical reviews of this literature have been reported by Witelson (1977), McGlone (1980), Bryden (1981), and McKeever (1981) and, for this reason, only a few brief comments will be made here. Most reviews concur in their evaluation of the developmental literature—namely, that the evidence is weak, at best, for positing a sex difference in hemispheric speech organization in children. This conclusion, if correct, again presents serious conceptual problems for those proponents of a sex difference in adolescents and adults. However, such conceptual issues may not have to be confronted when one examines critically the adult literature. The evidence again is weak. Both Bryden (1981) and McKeever (1981) have shown that extraneous strategy and scanning effects in the auditory and visual laterality studies can influence the direction and degree of laterality scores. In fact, Bryden (1981) has shown that the sex differences disappear when extraneous variance is more controlled. An additional problem with these behavioral approaches is the issue of reliability and validity (Satz, 1977). Many dichotic listening and visual half-field studies report verbal laterality advantages that depart significantly from the known incidence of left-hemisphere speech in right-handers. Not infrequently, only a slight majority of right-handers show the expected right-ear advantage (REA) or right visual half-field advantage (RVHF) on these tasks. In such instances, inferences to hemispheric speech specialization are invalid, as Satz (1977) has already demonstrated. Failure to control for familial handedness is another of the many factors that can also bias the direction and magnitude of the laterality advantages (Bryden, 1981; McKeever, 1981).

The largest study to date showing sex differences in the cerebral specialization of speech was conducted by Bryden (1976). He administered a dichotic consonant–vowel (CV syllables) tape to 72 normal left-handers (36 male, 36 female) and to 72 normal right-handers (36 male, 36 female). Although no effects of handedness were found, which raises serious questions concerning the validity of his task, Bryden did observe a larger laterality effect in the males, regardless of handedness group. This effect was also seen when the data were analyzed in terms of the frequency of laterality advantages. Within right-handers, 83% of the males ($p < .05$) and only 61% of the females ($p > .10$) showed a REA. Within left-handers, 67% of the males ($p < .05$) and only 56% of the females ($p > .10$) showed a REA.

Although Bryden (1976, 1981) has repeatedly recommended caution in interpreting these results, they have often been cited as evidence for sexual dimorphism in hemispheric functional specialization (McGlone, 1980). The major flaw in this conclusion is the fact that Bryden (1976) found no main effect of handedness on this dichotic task. It is now well established that the cerebral organization of speech is different in the left- and right-handed. Left-handers have been shown to have an increased probability of bilateral hemispheric speech representation (Gloning & Quatember, 1966; Hecaen & Sauquet, 1971; Milner, 1973; Satz, 1979; Hochberg & LeMay, 1977). Furthermore, although the males in Bryden's (1976) study showed a higher proportion of REAs, the females also showed a similar directional advantage; this overlap in REAs strongly counters claims of an underlying dimorphism in lateralization.

More serious concerns could be raised when one examines the stability of this perceptual asymmetry across studies. In Bryden's (1979) review, one finds far more negative than positive reports of a sex difference. Where positive results have been reported, the differences have been small with much overlap between gender groups, and the sample sizes have also been quite small.

In a recent study in our laboratory, we reexamined the issue of sex differences in perceptual asymmetries using the largest sample of sex differences in perceptual asymmetries using the largest sample of left- and right-handed males and females yet reported. In the study, 300 left-handers (male = 112, female = 188) and 221 right-handers (male = 84, female = 136) were administered a three-pair, computer-generated, dichotic word tape. This particular tape, using a free recall condition, has been shown to produce highly reliable REAs in the right-handed (Fennell, Bowers, & Satz, 1977; L. Costa, personal communication). Similar results were observed in the present study: 86% of the right-handers showed a REA. Of particular note was the finding that the REA proportions were virtually identical between gender groups, regardless of handedness.

In sum, we were unable to find any evidence of a sex difference on this laterality measure or on any of the other laterality measures employed. This finding provides additional evidence against the sexual dimorphism/laterality hypothesis. It was already shown that the hypothesis suffers on conceptual grounds; its empirical support seems equally weak. Although McGlone (1980) has argued that the hypothesis provides a parsimonious explanation of sex–brain differences in lateralization, Kinsbourne (1980) has correctly noted that this explanation confuses "parsimonious" with "simplistic." Kinsbourne states that "it is simplistic but not parsimonious to postulate a new phenomenon when our existing knowledge of relevant variables has not been fully used in our attempt to account conservatively for the phenomenon in question [p. 242]."

Given the concerns raised in this review, one might ask why the hypothesis continues to enjoy such widespread acceptance in the literature. Kinsbourne (1980) provides one account:

> Because the study of sex differences is not like the rest of psychology. Under pressure from the gathering momentum of feminism, and perhaps in backlash to it, many investigators seem determined to discover that men and women "really" are different. It seems that if sex differences (e.g., in lateralization) do not exist, then they have to be invented [p. 242].

SEX DIFFERENCES IN ATTACK RATES OF SPEECH AND LANGUAGE DISORDERS

The preceding sections have examined some of the prevailing views on sex-related differences in cognitive abilities and hemispheric specialization and have found them to be wanting on both conceptual and methodological grounds. Although the evidence is less clear regarding a male advantage in spatial visualization ability, the differences found have been neither robust nor reliable enough to warrant claims of a biological dimorphism on these traits. At best, one might merely conclude that sex represents a variable that accounts for a small proportion of the variance on the measured trait (i.e., spatial visualization). Given this state of affairs, one can understand why the search for biological substrates of these cognitive differences has been unrewarding. The construct, namely, hemispheric specialization, has suffered at both conceptual and methodological levels. It is for this reason that we choose to call these positions myths. They have misled us more than they have informed us. And they have provided no useful framework for understanding the causes, course, or prognosis of speech and language disorders in children.

The purpose of this final section is to suggest that we address the problem of sex differences from a different perspective, free of the controversy, bias, and dogma associated with the approaches that we have discussed. The approach we have in mind is to put aside further speculations on the presence and nature of sex-related cognitive differences in *normal* development and confront directly the issue of known sex differences in the attack rates in *abnormal* development—especially the various speech and language disorders.

A review of this literature reveals a higher incidence of males in each of the developmental disorders of speech and language. The sex ratios across the various disorders show a striking similarity, as can be seen in Table 6.1. A sex ratio of approximately 4 to 1, favoring males, can be seen for infantile autism, delayed speech, developmental dyslexia, and stuttering. In contrast to findings reported in previous sections of this chapter, these sex ratios are remarkably consistent across studies.

What clues, if any, do these differential sex ratios provide us with? In and of themselves, they tell us little; one must seek to understand the basis for these differences. It has been suggested that these differential attack rates represent a vulnerability that is higher in males and which lowers their mortality and morbidity thresholds throughout the life cycle (Taylor & Ounsted, 1972; Bentzen, 1963). Although males predominate at conception (approximately 130:100),

TABLE 6.1
Sex Ratios and Prevalences for the Developmental Language Disorders[a]

	Male–female ratio	Approximate prevalence (per 10,000 children)
Infantile autism	3.8/1	1
Delayed speech	4.0/1	60
Developmental dyslexia	3.5/1	500
Stuttering	3.8/1	70

[a]Based on data reported by Hier and Kaplan (1980).

this ratio decreases at birth (approximately 110:100) reflecting an increased morbidity during pregnancy (Masland, Sarason, & Gladwin, 1958). In fact, throughout pregnancy, the losses due to abortion, miscarriage, and stillbirth are consistently greater for males (Taylor & Ounsted, 1972). Potter and Adair (1946) showed that 78% of the stillborn fetuses delivered before the fourth month are male. Pasamanick (1960) reported a higher incidence of fetal and neonatal death rates as well as stillbirth rates for males; moreover, throughout life, males are reported to show higher morbidity rates due to brain injury.

The higher incidence in males of stillbirths and of death and disease during the first year of life has been cited as evidence of the greater vulnerability of the male organism to stress and trauma.[3] This vulnerability is further expressed in the overrepresentation of males in most disease states throughout the life cycle, including disorders of speech and language. Males are usually the more susceptible or at lower thresholds for expressing the disorder.

Why is this the case? Taylor and Ounsted (1972) have advanced an intriguing ontogenetic explanation for these sex differences in attack rates, morbidity, and mortality. Briefly, they postulate a difference in maturation rate which is presumed to be slower in males, thus prolonging their period of risk or vulnerability during the critical early developmental periods.

> Males develop more slowly than females, they delay their development in a wide variety of systems. In so doing they are more exposed to any risks attendant upon that developmental delay (such as febrile convulsions) and as compared to girls will be over-represented in any sampling in which the characteristic is fundamentally related to developmental pace (such as reading disorders). . . . Delay in development affords more opportunity to interact with the environment in a less mature state and this implies that more information may be derived from the genome, some of which may be disadvantageous. The delay in the emergence of the characteristic suggests that the variance of that characteristic for males will be greater than that for females. Relatively more males will be represented at the extreme of the spread of the characteristic. Where this crosses the threshold into the pathological area, although boys will be more numerous than girls, the girls will have required a relatively greater degree of divergence from their norm and hence will be the "worse" affected [pp. 231–232].

This position, while admittedly speculative, provides an intriguing explanation for the overrepresentation of males, particularly in the speech and language disorders. More difficult to follow is the prediction of an interaction between sex and severity level. Empirical support for this hypothesis stems from Taylor and Ounsted's (1972) ontogenetic analysis of the epilepsies. They report that in convulsions associated with fever, boys are more often affected but that morbid sequelae are relatively more common in girls. The basis for this explanation

---

[3]Note that this position does not imply a sexual dimorphism in morbidity or vulnerability; it merely states that males in general are at greater risk for these outcomes but that some females and not all males may be so disposed.

apparently relates to peak onset time (and decline) of seizures triggered by fever. They found that peak onset and timing of the decline comes earlier in females: "In general the earlier the age of onset of the convlusions the worse the prognosis. Since females are relatively over-represented in the early onset groups they are relatively more likely to suffer a serious outcome [p. 221]."

Our purpose in presenting this viewpoint is to raise a number of questions that may ultimately provide new approaches and, hopefully, some answers regarding the causes, course, and prognosis of speech and language disorders in children. Despite the controversy that studies of sex differences have engendered, the existence of differential attack rates still remains to be explained. The hypothesis of delayed maturation and prolonged risk vulnerability in males (Taylor & Ounsted, 1972) is an intriguing explanation that has some empirical support in the literature. Of even greater interest are the issues it raises concerning peak onset and decline periods of risk as they relate to symptom severity and prognosis in the various speech and language disorders. These questions have seldom been asked, mainly because of the overrepresentation of males in most of the clinical studies. The few female index cases ascertained have often been pooled with the males or excluded from study. For example, in the Florida Longitudinal Project (Fletcher & Satz, 1982), only white males from two large kindergarten populations were selcted in the prospective study of developmental dyslexia. Similar subject selection procedures have also been used in many of the longitudinal and cross-sectional studies of autism, developmental aphasia, and stuttering.

If the attack rates for these disorders are higher in males, as the literature strongly suggests, then males must have a lower threshold of liability, regardless of etiology. Conversely, females would be predicted to have a higher threshold of liability.

Given this premise, one might then ask whether the higher threshold of liability in females is associated with gender differences in onset of symptoms, severity level, and pattern and course of the disorder. According to Taylor and Ounsted (1972), females with febrile convulsions would be expected to have an earlier onset of symptoms with more severe sequelae, although males would be overrepresented in the cohort. Unfortunately, we do not know whether this finding, if true, would generalize to other developmental disorders. With respect to speech and language disorders, we do not know whether the peak onset of symptoms occurs earlier in females. If it does, is it related to symptom severity level, pattern of information-processing ability, or prognosis? These are questions that deserve further study.

Some information is available concerning prognosis as well as severity of symptoms at referral. A few longitudinal studies (Bruck, 1981; Peter & Spreen, 1979: Werner & Smith, 1977) have pointed to more severe sequelae in girls with learning disorders. The Peter and Spreen (1979) study showed that females referred with learning handicap between the ages of 8 to 14 had significantly higher scores (greater impairment) during late adolescence than males on all four scales of a self-report adjustment inventory (home, health, social, and emotional adjustments) as well as on five out of six indices of socioemotional adjustment as rated by the parents. Further analyses indicated that the differences obtained were not due to sex differences in sample size, or to a sex-related bias in response to the scales. Also, at initial referral there were no apparent sex differences in demographic variables such as socioeconomic status and intelligence level. In fact, the differences in later adjustment held for groups of equal numbers of males and females matched for age, IQ, and degree of neurological impairment.

The Peter and Spreen findings suggest that while socioemotional prognosis is worse in a heterogenous group of learning-disordered girls, the severity of cognitive difficulty at initial referral is not different from the boys, at least as measured by IQ or degree of neurological impairment. Decker and DeFries (1980), using a more homogenous learning-disabled sample, found that boys and girls were equally impaired in reading. Finucci and Childs (1981) reported that the most severe reading disability occurred among their male cohorts and that there were fewer females at every level of reading impairment except the most mild. Bryan and Pflaun (1978) examined the linguistic performance of a group of 10- to 11-year-old male and female learning-disabled children. They found that the male cohorts used significantly less complex social communications than nondisabled same-sex peers. However, no linguistic differences were found between the learning-disabled and nondisabled females. Taken together, these findings suggest that when a female is affected by a learning disorder or a reading difficulty she will be no more severely impaired than a male and is, in fact, more likely to be superior with respect to linguistic performance or reading.

How, then, do we reconcile the consistent findings of poorer emotional outcome in females with their equal or better cognitive performance at referral? The analogy with the developmental disorders discussed by Taylor and Ounsted (1972) lacks several components: For example, in language disorders little is known about sex differences in age of peak onset. Nevertheless, Taylor and Ounsted's analysis may be invoked to account for the relatively poor sequelae in females. First, following their logic, it may be assumed that when a girl acquires the disorder it represents a relatively greater divergence from the norm for girls. In other words, when girls have a learning problem it is more likely to reflect the presence of biological risk factors which may lead to more severe sequelae. This type of notion is consistent with DeFries and Decker's finding that a greater proportion of the relatives of reading-disabled girls are affected than reading-disabled boys. That is, for females to be reading disabled they must have a greater genetic loading (i.e., more "risk" genes) than disabled males. A similar observation was made by Kidd, Kidd, and Records (1978) for female stutterers. The possibility of a greater genetic loading factor in affected females would point to a greater severity of symptoms relative to males. Much of the evidence reviewed, however, indicates that such is not the case. There is no contradiction, however, if it is assumed that the loading factor pushes the female toward a pathological extreme relative to the *female* norm.

A second possibility has sociocultural roots. If girls with reading disability are more atypical or unexpected they may be perceived or treated in ways which would make later adjustment worse. For example, girls may not be referred as readily thus allowing the problem to go untreated for longer periods; or their deviance from cultural expectation may not be as acceptable as male deviance. Few studies have systematically compared learning-disabled boys and girls with respect to emotional disposition, but prevailing knowledge indicates a greater degree of asocial behavior in affected males. It is therefore difficult, at this level, to ascribe the reported differences in later adjustment to early patterns of emotional functioning.

Another type of factor stems from the possibility that any language disorder may have several different causes any of which could vary systematically as a function of gender and which may result in different outcomes. For example, the later status of reading-disabled boys and girls matched on IQ, reading level, and other relevant demographic variables may differ because of differences in patterns of neuropsychological functioning. However, a report by Canning, Orr, and Rourke (1981) found no such differences in two age groups of learning-disabled children.

In an ongoing analysis of three different samples of learning-disordered children in Victoria, referred either to school evaluation centers or to the university clinic, we noted a remarkably consistent pattern: Girls had IQ scores lower than boys by amounts greater than would be expected in nonclinic samples (Kaufman & Doppelt, 1976). At the same time the girls' scores in reading and spelling relative to their IQ levels were significantly better than the boys'. Closer examination of the data indicated that for a majority of the girls the learning problems stemmed from overall low functioning in verbal and visuospatial areas, whereas in a majority of the boys the problem was one of specific learning retardation. Moreover, as seen in other studies, the severity of the reading difficulty in those boys with specific reading problems (IQs in the normal range) was not different from the degree of the reading difficulty in the relatively small number of girls with specific reading problems. What these recent observations suggest is that for girls referred with learning problems there may be a greater probability of later difficulty because they are more severely impaired in terms of surrounding factors associated with the difficulty, rather than specific processes directly involved in the production of the difficulty. Other data, referred to earlier, suggest, however, that even in that subset of learning-disabled girls in which surrounding factors are apparently similar to boys', girls will still be at a disadvantage at outcome, because pathological factors (i.e., increased genetic loading) have pushed them into a particular state of vulnerability and/or because of sociocultural attitudes that are brought to bear on the atypical female. It is clear that at present the data do not permit firm conclusions. With respect to our own pilot data one might well ask whether there is a referral bias at work. Are females more likely to be referred when their academic difficulty is associated with other problems or is it in fact the case that females are more likely to be likely to be learning handicapped for reasons associated with more general cognitive problems? Questions such as these are currently being addressed.[4]

This chapter, in summary, has examined a number of issues on sex differences in both normal and abnormal development. Some myths have been exposed and some clues for future research have been suggested. The clues have been presented in the spirit of questions rather than formal hypotheses. They may in time prove untenable. Hopefully, they will at least be heuristic.

ACKNOWLEDGMENT

The comments of the NINCDS Task Force are gratefully acknowledged.

REFERENCES

Andrews, G., & Harris, M. M. *The syndrome of stuttering.* London: Heineman, 1964.
Bentzen, F. Sex ratios in learning and behavior disorders. *American Journal of Orthopsychiatry,* 1963, *33,*
Bryan & Plaun (1978)
Bryden, M. P. Response bias and hemispheric difference in dot localization. *Perceptual Psychophsiology,* 19, 23–28.
Bryden, M. P. Evidence for sex-related differences in cerebral organization. In M. A. Wittig & A. C. Peterson (Eds.), *Sex-related differences in cognitive functioning: Developmental issues.* New York: Academic Press, 1979.
Bryden, M. P. Sex-related differences in cerebral hemispheric asymmetry and their possible relation to dyslexia. In A. Ansara, N. Geschwind, A. Galaburda, M. Albert, & N. Gartrell (Eds.), *Sex differences in dyslexia.* Towson, Md.: Orton Dyslexia Society, 1981.
Buffery, A. W. H. & Gray, J. A. Sex differences in the development of spatial and linguistic skills. In C. Ounsted & D. C. Taylor (Eds.), *Gender differences: Their ontogeny and significance.* London: Churchill Livingstone, 1972.
Canning, P. M., Orr, R., & Rourke, B. P. Sex differences in the perceptual, visual–motor, linguistic and concept-formational abilities of retarded readers. *Journal of Learning Disabilities,* 1980, *13, 9,*
Canter, R., Hohenegger, M., & Satz, P. Handedness & aphasia: An inferential method for determining the mode of cerebral speech specialization. *Neuropsychologia,* 1980, *18,* 569–575.
Decker, J. C. & DeFries, S. N. Cognitive abilities in families with reading disabled children. *Journal of Learning Disabilities,* 1980, *13, 9,*
Dobzhansky, T. *Genetic diversity and human equality.* New York: Basic Books, 1973.
Fairweather, H. Sex differences in cognition. *Cognition,* 1976, *4,* 231–280.

---

[4]The interested reader might benefit from a review of the literature on sex differences in schizophrenia (Lewine, 1981). Although the attack rates are similar in males and females, studies have consistently revealed an earlier onset of symptoms and first hospitalization for schizophrenia in males along with a more typical symptom picture and poorer premorbid social competence. Although both biological and environmental explanations have been advanced to account for these differences, the evidence, as with speech and language disorders, remains unclear.

Fennell, E. B., Bowers, D., & Satz, P. Within modal and cross-modal reliabilities of two laterality tests. *Brain and Language,* 1977, *4,* 63–69.

Finucci, M. J., & Childs, B. Are there really more dyslexic boys than girls? In A. Ansara, N. Geschwind, A. Galaburda, M. Albert & N. Gartrell (Eds.), *Sex differences in dyslexia.* Towson, Md.: Orton Dyslexia Society, 1981.

Fletcher, J., Satz, P., & Morris, R. Florida Longitudinal Project: A review. In S. Mednick & M. Harway (Eds.), *Longitudinal research.* New York: Oxford University Press, 1981. (a)

Fletcher, J., Satz, P., & Morris, R. The Florida Longitudinal Project: Theoretical implications. In S. A. Mednick & M. A. Harway (Eds.), *U.S. longitudinal projects.* New York: Cambridge University Press, 1981. (b)

Fox, L. H., Tobin, D., & Brady, L. Sex role socialization and achievement in mathematics. In M. A. Wittig & A. C. Petersen (Eds.), *Sex-related differences in cognitive functioning: Developmental issues.* New York: Academic Press, 1979.

Gloning, I., & Quatember, R. Statistical evidence of neuropsychological syndrome in left-handed and ambidextrous patients. *Cortex,* 1966, *2,* 484–488.

Hacaen, H., & Sauquet, J. Cerebral dominance in left-handed subjects. *Cortex,* 1971, *7,* 19–48.

Hier, D. B., & Kaplan, J. Are sex differences in cerebral organization clinically significant? *The Behavioral and Brain Sciences,* 1980, *3,* 238–239.

Hochberg, F. H., & LeMay, M. Asymmetries of the skull and handedness. *Journal of Neurological Science,* 1977, *32,* 243–253.

Inglis, J., & Lawson, J. S. Sex differences in the effects of unilateral brain damage on intelligence. *Science,* 1981, *212,* 693–695.

Jacklin, C. N. Epilogue. In M. A. Wittig & A. C. Petersen (Eds.), *Sex-related differences in cognitive functioning: Developmental issues.* New York: Academic Press, 1979.

Kaufman, A. S., & Doppelt, J. E. Analyses of WISC-R standardization data in terms of the stratification variables. *Child Development,* 1976, *47,* 165–171.

Kertesz, A. Are there sex differences in acquired aphasia? In A. Ansara, N. Geschwind, A. Galaburda, M. Albert, & N. Gartrell (Eds.), *Sex differences in dyslexia.* Towson, Md.: Orton Dyslexia Society, 1981.

Kertesz, A. & Sheppard. The epidemology of aphasic and cognitive impairment in stroke: Age, sex, aphasia type and laterality differences. *Brain,* 1981, *104,* 117–128.

Kidd, K. K., Kidd, J. R., & Records, M. A. On possible causes of the sex ratio in stuttering and its implications. *Journal of Fluency Disorders,* 1978, *3,* 13–23.

Kinsbourne, M. If sex differences in brain lateralization exist, they have yet to be discovered. Cited in J. McGlone, Sex differences in human brain asymmetry: A critical survey. *The Behavioral and Brain Sciences,* 1980, *3,* 215–263.

Kinsbourne, M., & Hiscock, M. Does cerebral dominance develop? In S. Segalowitz & F. Gruber (Eds.), *Language development and neurological theory.* New York: Academic Press, 1977.

Lansdell, H. A sex difference in effect of temporal lobe neurosurgery on design preference. *Nature,* 1962, *194,* 852–854.

Lansdell, H. Effect of extent of temporal lobe ablations on two lateralized deficits. *Physiology and Behavior,* 1968, *3,* 271–273.

Lansdell, H., & Urbach, N. Sex differences in personality measures related to size and side of temporal lobe ablations. *Proceedings of the 73rd Annual Convention of the APA,* 1965, 113–114.

Maccoby, E. E., & Jacklin, C. N. *The psychology of sex differences.* Stanford: Stanford University Press, 1974.

Marshall, W. A., & Tanner, M. Variations in the pattern of pubertal change in boys. *Archives of Disease in Childhood,* 1970, *45,* 13–23.

Masland, R. L., Sarason, S. B., & Gladwin, T. *Mental subnormality.* New York: Basic Books, 1958.

Matarazzo, J. D. *Wechsler's measurement and appraisal of adult intelligence.* Baltimore, Md.: Williams and Wilkins, 1972.

McGlone, J. Sex differences in human brain asymmetry: A critical survey. *The Behavioral and Brain Sciences,* 1980, *3,* 215–263.

McGlone, J. Sex differences in the cerebral organization of verbal functions in patients with unilateral brain lesions. *Research Bulletin,* No. 399, ISSN 0316–4675, Univ. Western Ontario, 1976.

McGlone, J. Sex differences in functional brain asymmetry. *Cortex,* 1978, *14,* 122–128.

McGlone, J., & Kertesz, A. Sex differences in cerebral processing of visuo-spatial tasks. *Cortex,* 1973, *9,* 313–320.

McGlone, J., & Kertesz, A. Sex differences in cerebral processing of visuo-spatial tasks. *Cortex,* 1973, *9,* 313–320.

McKeever, W. F. Sex and cerebral organization: Is it really so simple? In A. Ansara, N. Geschwind, A. Galaburda, M. Albert, & N. Gartrell (Eds.), *Sex differences in dyslexia.* Towson, Md.: Orton Dyslexia Society, 1981.

Meyer, V., & Jones, H. Patterns of cognitive tests performance as functions of lateral localization of cerebral abnormalities in the temporal lobe. *Journal of Mental Science,* 1957, *103,* 758–772.

Milner, B. *Effects of early left hemisphere lesions on cerebral organization of function in man.* Paper presented at the annual meeting of the American Psychological Association, New Orleans, 1973.

Morgan, M. J. Influences of sex on variation in human brain asymmetry. Cited in J. McGlone, Sex differences in human brain asymmetry; A critical survey. *The Behavioral and Brain Sciences,* 1980, *3,* 215–263.

Nash, S. C. Sex role as a mediator of intellectual functioning. In M. A. Wittig & A. C. Petersen (Eds.), *Sex-related differences in cognitive functioning: Developmental issues.* New York: Academic Press, 1979.

Pasamanick, B. Personal communication, November 1, 1960, to F. Bentzen, Sex ratios in learning and behavior disorders. *American Journal of Orthopsychiatry,* 1963, *33,* 92–98.

Peter, B. M., & Spreen, O. Behavior rating and personal adjustment scales of neurologically and learning handicapped children during adolescence and early adulthood: Results of a follow-up study. *Journal of Clinical Neuropsychology,* 1979, *1,* 75–92.

Petersen, A. C. Hormones and cognitive functioning in normal development. In M. A. Wittig & A. C. Petersen (Eds.), *Sex-related differences in cognitive functioning: Developmental issues.* New York: Academic Press, 1979.

Petersen, A. C. Sex differences in performance on spatial tasks: Biopsychosocial influences. In A. Ansara, N. Geschwind, A. Galaburda, M. Alpert, & N. Gartrell (Eds.), *Sex differences in dyslexia.* Towson, Md.: Orton Dyslexia Society, 1981.

Potter, E. L., & Adair, F. *Fetal and neo-natal death.* Chicago: University of Chicago Press, 1946.

Satz, P. Cerebral dominance and reading disability: An old problem revisited. In R. Knights & P. J. Bakker (Eds.), *The neuropsychology of learning disorders: Theoretical approaches* (Proceedings of NATA conference). Baltimore, Md.: University Park Press, 1976.

Satz, P. Laterality tasks: An inferential problem. *Cortex,* 1977, *13,* 208–212.

Satz, P. A test of some models of hemispheric speech organization in the left- and right-handed. *Science,* 1979, *203,* 1131–1133.

Satz, P. Incidence of aphasia in left-handers: A test of some hypothetical models of cerebral speech organization. In J. Herron (Ed.), *The neuropsychology of left-handedness.* New York: Academic Press, 1980.

Satz, P., & Bullard-Bates, C. Acquired aphasia in children. In M. T. Sarno (Ed.), *Acquired aphasia.* New York: Academic Press, 1981.

Taylor, D. C., & Ounsted, C. *The nature of gender differences explored through ontogenetic analyses of sex ratios in disease.* Unpublished manuscript, 1972.

Tobach, E. The meaning of cryptanthroparion. In L. Ehrman, G. S. Omenn, & E. Caspari (Eds.), *Genetics, environment and behavior.* New York: Academic Press, 1972.

Waber, D. P. Differences in cognitive functioning: Developmental sex differences in cognition—A function of maturation rate? *Science,* 1976, *192,* 572–574.

Waber, D. P. Sex differences in mental abilities, hemispheric lateralization, and rate of physical growth at adolescence. *Developmental Psychology,* 1977, *13,* 29–38.

Waber, D. P. Cognitive abilities and sex-related variations in the maturation of cerebral cortical functions. In M. A. Wittig & A. C. Petersen (Eds.), *Sex-related differences in cognitive functioning: Developmental issues.* New York: Academic Press, 1979.

Werner, E. E., & Smith, R. S. *Kanai's children come of age.* Honolulu: University Press of Hawaii, 1977.

Wittig, M. A. Genetic influences on sex-related differences in intellectual performance: Theoretical and methodological issues. In M. A. Wittig & A. C. Petersen (Eds.), *Sex-related differences in cognitive functioning: Developmental issues.* New York: Academic Press, 1979.

Wittig, M. A., & Petersen, A. C. Sex-related differences in cognitive functioning: An overview. In M. A. Wittig & A. C. Petersen (Eds.), *Sex-related differences in cognitive functioning: Developmental issues.* New York: Academic Press, 1979.

Witelson, S. F. Sex and the single hemisphere: Specialization of the right hemisphere for spatial processing. *Science,* 1976, *193,* 425–427.

Witelson, S. F. Developmental dyslexia: Two right hemispheres and no left? *Science,* 1977, *195,* 309–311.

Woods, B. T., & Teuber, H. L. Changing patterns of childhood aphasia. *Transactions of the American Neurological Association,* 1977, *102,* 36–38.

Zurif, E. B., & Carson, G. Dyslexia in relation to cerebral and temporal analysis. *Neuropsychologia,* 1970, *8,* 351–361.

III

INVESTIGATION OF GENOTYPE: METHODOLOGY AND RESEARCH DESIGNS

7

Twin Studies and the Etiology of Complex Neurological Disorders

ROSWELL ELDRIDGE

INTRODUCTION

The study of twins can provide basic understanding of complex traits or disorders through a number of approaches. Among these approaches are the following: determination of heritability, as has been applied to intelligence (Jensen, 1970); defining discrete subgroups within heterogeneous disorders, as has been applied to diabetes mellitus (Rotter & Rimoin, 1978) and peptic ulcer disease (Rotter, 1980); separating maternal factors from other environmental influences (Nance, 1979); suggesting precipitating factors through prospective study of unaffected co-twins; and seeking etiologic clues through retrospective case control studies.

It is the first approach—that is, the determination of the heritability (or contribution to the variance due to genetic factors)—that most associate with twin studies. But in recent years this use has been seriously questioned, largely because the tendency has been to extrapolate findings from the study of highly selected twin pairs to the general population. The biologic limitations of the twin method and the inherent bias in ascertainment of twin "volunteers" have often not been given sufficient weight.

On the other hand, the last approach, which seeks clues as to etiology through use of twins by the "case control" method, should be useful in disorders in which genetic and environmental factors appear to play a role. Thus, the complex and no doubt heterogeneous disorders that are the subject of this book, certainly should benefit from this approach.

One obvious advantage of the use of twins as case controls is the reduction

109

GENETIC ASPECTS OF
SPEECH AND LANGUAGE DISORDERS

ISBN 0–12–459350–X

in variables, both genetic and environmental. Some of these variables are presented at Table 7.1, Part A, which also indicates other advantages of the approach. For those embarking on a study of relatively unexplored areas, such as that of speech and language disorders, the fact that the subtle differences, or risk factors, are often detectable, the low cost of such studies, and the high degree of motivation of the participating twins can prove particularly important.

Equally important are the very real limitations or weaknesses of this approach. Some of these are listed in Part B of the table. Particularly relevant for any trait involving communication is the unique relationship between twins and the effect this has on "normal" language development. However, study of pairs discordant for the communicative disorders should still be productive. The large population needed to generate sufficient twin pairs should not be an obstacle in studying conditions as prevalent among youth as those under discussion. Given that in the United States approximately 1% of the population are twins, and that the prevalance of speech disorders alone varies from 10–15% in children of ages 6–7 to 1–2% in youths aged 17 (Leske, 1981), there is little question that an adequate number of twin pairs exists in this segment of the population which is said to number over 2 million (Leske, 1981). Whether such pairs can be marshaled for study and whether an appropriate multidisciplinary task force can be assembled is another matter. Regarding the first point, if a specific factor or event is associated with a fourfold increase in risk, there is a 99% probability of its demonstration if 50 discordant twin pairs are available for matched analysis. If the relative risk is only 2, matched analyses of 100 discor-

TABLE 7.1
"Case Control" Twin Studies[a]

A. Strengths
  1. MZs and DZs are automatically matched for a number of factors: age; geographic setting of birth; birth cohort; birth order; parental age; ethnic and cultural heritage; childhood social class, education, and medical care; understanding intent of questions.
  2. MZs have nearly identical genome, including HLA haplotypes.
  3. Subtle differences between twins are often detectable.
  4. Motivation is generally high in co-twin.
  5. Both concordant and discordant pairs are valuable.
  6. Young MZ twins, discordant for disorder, are at increased risk.
  7. Cost is low.
B. Weaknesses or limitations
  1. Large population is needed.
  2. Bias in twin volunteers.
  3. Twins differ from singletons:
     in utero: placentation, circulation, shared surroundings
     at birth: often premature; second born has longer labor
     in youth: twin–twin relationship
  4. Co-twin is at risk for uncertain period.
  5. Co-twin may have subclinical disease.

[a]Modified from Mack, 1981.

TABLE 7.2
Power of Matched Analysis, Case-Control Studies[a] ($p \leq .05$)

	Relative risk		
Number of discordant pairs	1.5	2.0	4.0
20	.16	.34	.85
50	.35	.73	.99
100	.60	.98	.99
200	.87	.99	.99

[a]Theoretical analyses cited by Thomas Mack, personal communication, 1981.

dant pairs will still demonstrate such an association with a 98% probability (Table 7.2).

A critical issue that must be resolved early in the planning of a twin study concerns its scope. The range of questions that can be addressed has already been indicated. Obviously, not all of these questions can or should be dealt with in a single study. On the other hand, the opportunity to interview and examine a large sample of twins occurs rarely so the inclination is to cover as much ground as possible. The feat, as can be seen in the projects described in what follows, is not to tackle too much.

In the remainder of this chapter I describe twin studies with multiple sclerosis (MS) and Parkinson's disease (PD). Emphasis is placed on methods of ascertainment and determination of concordance status. Also included are the results of certain "opportunistic" studies that sought to take advantage of the twin phenomenon. Pitfalls encountered along the often torturous way are described in considerable detail in hopes of sparing those readers who are considering taking the same path.

TWIN STUDIES IN MULTIPLE SCLEROSIS

This neurological disorder is characterized clinically by a variety of neurological deficits "separated in time and space," with onset generally between the ages of 20 and 50. The course is generally relapsing and remitting, but there is great variability. Although there is general agreement as to criteria for diagnosis of MS and classification of clinical stages, there is no laboratory test that is diagnostic. Ultimate confirmation rests upon autopsy which reveals multiple discrete plagues scattered throughout the white matter of the central nervous system.

For the past 5 years a multidisciplinary study of twins has been in progress in our institution. The study evolved from a collaborative investigation of "familial MS" which clearly indicated that a single mutant gene was not responsible for the disorder (Eldridge, McFarland, Sever, Sadowsky, & Krebs, 1978). We now have completed study of 51 selected twin pairs. In what follows, the question of heritability is addressed by comparison of concordance rates in monozygotic and dizygotic twins, and possible risk factors are considered through use of a preliminary case control study (Currier & Eldridge, 1981). Clinical and laboratory findings based on 30 twin pairs are described (Williams, Eldridge, McFarland, Houff, Krebs, & McFarlin, 1980). Finally, immunogenetic observations on a small sample of twins are discussed (Eldridge, McFarlin, & McFarland, 1982).

Ascertainment

To date, over 140 twin pairs have been ascertained, primarily through notice in the *MS Messenger,* the newsletter of the Multiple Sclerosis Society of the United States. Additional pairs were obtained through notices in medical and neurological journals, as well as through contact with medical colleagues and lay individuals.

Medical records were obtained, and those pairs in which at least one twin fulfilled the diagnostic criteria of Schumacher *et al.* (1965) were contracted. Those pairs in which both twins were available for study were personally evaluated, either at the Clinical Center, National Institutes of Health, where they were examined independently by three neurologists, or during home visits where they were examined by an experienced colleague (Robert D. Currier).

Genetic Epidemiology

An initial analysis has been conducted in 51 twin pairs (Currier & Eldridge, 1981). Figure 7.1 presents these 51 pairs, indicating zygosity, concordance, duration of disease, sex, birth order, and family history. Note the higher concordance in MZ twins. Lack of complete concordance in MZ twins over 50, beyond which age it is unlikely that one will develop MS, indicates that environmental factors play some role as well. Note also that of the 11 twin pairs concordant for MS, all are female. The implication is that genetic factors play a greater role in females. This is important because, if true, the etiology of MS is somewhat different in the two sexes. Therefore, results of any clinical MS study should be separated clearly according to sex. Emerging from a preliminary case control study, based on a detailed medical interview of these 102 twins by the same medical examiner, is the suggestion that certain events occurring in childhood through early adult life influence the risk for MS (Currier & Eldridge, 1982). These events consist of birth anoxia, serious infectious diseases during childhood or adolescence, multiple childbirth, and major operations. Although the association between these events and MS is significant at a level of p is equal to .05 or less, it is necessary to seek confirmation in a larger study of twins and

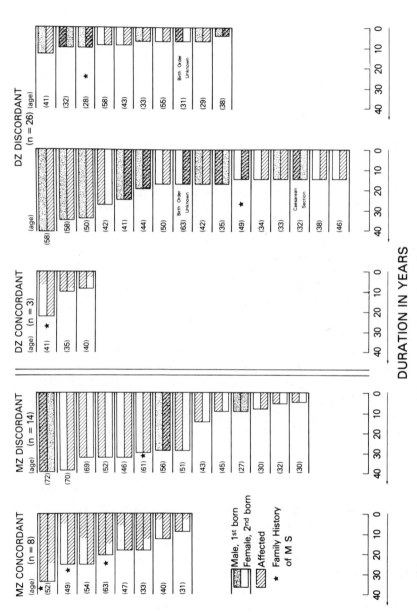

FIGURE 7.1. MS in 51 twin pairs by zygosity, concordance, duration, sex, birth order, and family history.

nontwins. If correct, to the extent these events can be modified, the risk for MS in susceptible individuals can be reduced.

Clinical and Laboratory Evaluation of Selected Twin Pairs

Thirty twin pairs, including 24 pairs from the preceding phase of the study, had extensive clinical, laboratory, and immune function evaluation at the National Institutes of Health Clinical Center. Clinical evaluation was performed independently by three neurologists. Zygosity was assessed on a clinical basis and then confirmed by standard genotyping as well as HLA determination. Genotyping and HLA confirmed the clinical impression for all but one twin pair. The exception was a female, MZ pair, in which one twin had had rhinoplasty and had dyed her hair. Several of the examiners in this instance failed to inquire whether these twins had looked alike "as two peas in a pod" as children.

In only 24 of the 30 pairs could a firm clinical diagnosis be made for each twin. (The 24 were all included in the larger series already described.) In the other 6 twin pairs a conclusion regarding concordance for MS could not be reached. In 3 of these pairs the proband had definite or possible MS and the co-twin had either a history of neurological dysfunction or a finding on examination suggesting MS but insufficient to lead to definite diagnosis. All 3 of these unclassifiable twins had CSF abnormalities consisting of either elevated IgM or oligoclonal bands, or both. These findings strongly suggest the existence of a "subclinical" form of MS.

In addition, among the clinically discordant pairs, 12 of 15 normal twins were found to have similar CSF abnormalities. Because of these findings and because typical MS plaques of demylination have been described in clinically normal cases (Georgi, 1961), subclinical disease may be occurring in some clinically normal twins as well. Supporting this suspicion has been the recent development of definite MS in two twins classified as only possible MS 2 years ago.

Immunologic Evaluation

Monozygotic discordant twins beyond the age at risk are ideal subjects for assessing immunologic function in disease. Because a viral agent has been indicated as a possible etiology in MS, both humoral immunity and cell-mediated immunity to candidate agents have been evaluated. Survey of the serum and CSF antibody against 12 viruses failed to show significant differences between the affected and unaffected twins (McFarlin & Madden, 1983).

Study of cellular immunity against mumps, vaccinia, and measles using a lymphoproliferative assay revealed no major differences in the response to vaccinia and mumps. Three twin sets were encountered in which one individual responded dramatically to measles while the co-twin showed only the normal low response. In all three cases the responder was the twin with MS.

An *in vivo* therapeutic trial involving lymphocyte transfer is being performed in selected twin pairs. In recent years, abnormalities in lymphocyte subsets have received considerable emphasis in MS. It is believed that here are reduced numbers of suppressor T cells in the presence of active disease. An immunologic lesion of this type could theoretically be modified by the transfer of normal histocompatible suppressor cells. Twins provide an opportunity to evaluate this possibility.

In a pair of 58-year-old male MZ twins discordant for MS approximately 10 billion lymphocytes were removed from the normal twin and transferred into the twin with MS. No adverse reaction was observed, thus establishing the feasibility of this approach. Initially, there was a suggestion of limited clinical improvement but this was mild and transient. No changes in oligoclonal bands or CSF immunoglobulin content were seen.

Discussion

The twin studies in multiple sclerosis included genetic–epidemiologic studies in a large sample of twins, clinical–laboratory studies in a smaller hospitalized sample, and, finally, immunogenetic and management studies in selected twin pairs. Among the contributions these studies have made are the following: understanding the nosology and natural history of MS (subclinical or preclinical MS); noting possible risk factors, several of which can be modified (surgery and multiple childbirth); and perfecting techniques for immunologic evaluation and management.

These twins provide a valuable resource for future study. The younger, presently unaffected co-twins provide a useful sample for prospective epidemiologic study. Twin pairs concordant for MS may be utilized for controlled therapeutic trials. Older, clinically unaffected co-twins will be important to study by procedures that can demonstrate small, asymptomatic lesions as well as ultimately by postmortem examination.

TWIN STUDIES IN PARKINSON'S DISEASE

Support for the genetic epidemiologic findings in twins with MS has come recently from a study of similar design involving twins with PD.

Parkinson's disease is one form of parkinsonism, a syndrome characterized by the triad of resting tremor, difficulty in initiating movement, and rigidity. Numerous conditions can lead to parkinsonism including encephalitis such as that seen with the flu epidemic that occurred toward the end of the First World War, and intoxication with heavy metals such as manganese. The etiology of PD, however, is uncertain. One study of selected families has suggested an important genetic contribution (Kondo, Kurland, & Schull, 1973), but a more rigorous evaluation during which many family members were actually examined by a single investigator did not support this contention (Duvoisin, Gearling, Schweiger *et al.,* 1969).

Extraordinary has been the paucity of twins reported with this condition, there being none from the United States until a preliminary note in 1981 (Duvoisin, Eldridge, Williams, Nutt, & Calne, 1981). This section presents a summary of our findings based on study of 78 twin pairs (Ward, Duvoisin, Ince, Nutt, Eldridge, & Calne, 1983).

Ascertainment

Twin pairs in which one or both were said to have PD were sought through multiple sources. These included direct contact with colleagues, notices in medical journals, announcements at neurology meetings, advertisements in newsletters of three voluntary PD organizations, contact with directors of the Veterans' Twin Registry of the National Academy of Science and the Kaiser–Permanente Twin Registry of California, and direct inquiry of over 750 Parkinson patients followed at four neurology centers in the eastern United States.

A total of 169 twin pairs have been ascertained over the 4-year period ending in September 1981. By far the most productive source was advertising in newsletters of the voluntary organizations. Least productive were direct solicitations of members of the neurological communities. Initially, emphasis was placed on ascertainment of MZ twins only, but in the second phase of the study equal emphasis has been placed on interesting DZ twins.

Genetic Epidemiology

Of the 169 twin pairs ascertained, it has been possible for at least one member of the nationwide neurologic team to examine both twins in 77 pairs. Preliminary review of medical recrods suggested at least one twin in each of these 77 pairs did have PD. In fact, 17 pairs were rejected because neither twin had typical PD. In two of these pairs there was concordance for parkinsonism, but additional features and unusual natural history were not compatible with the diagnosis of PD. Of the 60 twin pairs in which the index case has typical PD, 42 were MZ and 18 DZ. The unusually high proportion of MZ pairs reflects the early emphasis on their ascertainment and evaluation.

Selected clinical and genetic features of the first 52 of these twin pairs are presented in Figure 7.2. Of the 34 MZ pairs in this group, only 1 was concordant for PD, and none of the 17 DZ pairs were concordant. There was no unusual predominance by sex and no relation to brith order or birth weight. There was no family history of PD in the single concordant MZ pair but a positive history was present in 8 MZ disconcordant pairs and in 3 DZ pairs. None of the 77 twin pairs evaluated was black and, only one pair among the 169 ascertained was

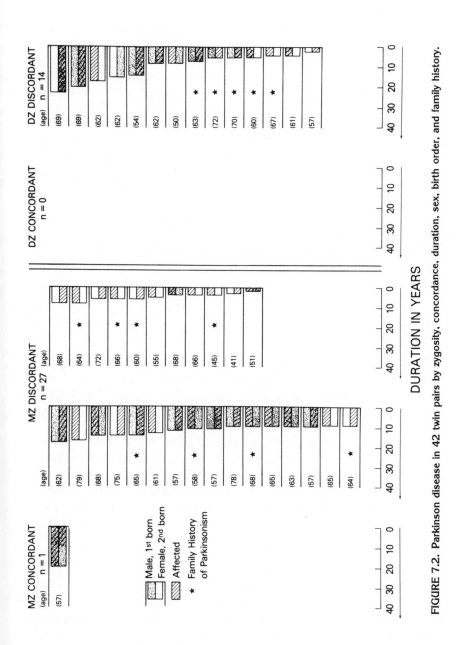

FIGURE 7.2. Parkinson disease in 42 twin pairs by zygosity, concordance, duration, sex, birth order, and family history.

black. This contrasts with the MS study in which 2 of the 24 pairs with MS studied at the National Institutes of Health were black.

At least one affected MZ twin (PD# 0056) among the discordant pairs had mild malformations. The affected member of pair #0056 was noted early in life to have her left leg slightly shorter and smaller than her right. Gait was affected and this permitted her parents to distinguish her from her co-twin, but it did not interfere with her social or athletic activities. About age 39 tremor present at rest developed in her left foot and soon was accompanied by symptoms suggesting bradykinesia, that is, slow or retarded movements. For several years the symptoms remained confined to the left leg but they then became noticeable in the left arm as well. When examined, at age 45, the left leg was one-half inch shorter than the right and one inch smaller in circumference at mid-thigh. The arms appeared symmetrical and no other dysmorphic change was noted. There was noticeable resting tremor and cogwheel rigidity of the left foot, ankle, and leg, with similar but less pronounced changes in the left arm. Mild but definite rigidity was present in the right arm as well but there was no tremor.

Hemiatrophy with hemi-parkinsonism is a recognized entity with onset in the fourth decade of life (Klawans, 1981). The parkinsonism is slowly progressive, but remains unilateral for 3–5 years, and the response to L-dopa is minimal. In the patient described here the malformation is mild and the disease, although asymmetric, has been progressive. The development of the initial symptom in the malformed limb in this discordant identical twin hardly seems coincidental.

The MZ twin pair concordant for PD were extremely similar in their medical histories as well as their developmental, social, academic, occupational, dietary, and geographic experiences. However, so, too, were at least 10 of the discordant MZ pairs, several of whom had shared the same domestic, academic, and occupational environment all their lives.

Several features did appear to distinguish some affected from nonaffected MZ twins. Preliminary analysis indicated the affected twin was usually the nonsmoker or the light smoker and was the more introverted and less dominant of the pair (Duvoisin, Eldridge, Williams, Nutt, & Calne, 1981). These differences have crucial implications for the timing and nature of the insult leading to PD but they require confirmation.

Discussion

The startling fact to emerge from this initial twin study of PD is the extraordinarily low concordance rate in both MZ and DZ twins. The rate is no higher in these twins than in the general population, which argues against either a major genetic contribution or a major environmental contribution as generally considered.

Ascertainment bias seems an unlikely explanation for such a low rate. The very different concordance rate found in the MS twin study, which shared similar ascertainment and design features, argues strongly that the concordance rates seen in each do indeed reflect the general concordance rates in the population, or at least in the twin population.

Clinical investigation of the twins did not identify a single environmental factor or event that determined the onset or course of PD in these twins. The suggestion that the personality differences observed tend to be lifelong and malformation influences distribution of symptoms support the notion that a predisposition to PD is acquired very early in life, possibly even in the prenatal period.

GENERAL RECOMMENDATIONS AND PITFALLS

Based on the experience that has been summarized here, acquired during study of over 200 twins having either MS or PD, the following comments are offered to those considering embarking on twin studies:

Realize at the outset that the findings in twins may not be applicable to the general "singleton" popuation. For a number of reasons, some of which are mentioned in Table 7.1, twins are unique.

If considering complex conditions for investigation, choose one in which there is good likelihood of ascertaining at least 100 twin pairs. As is illustrated in Table 7.2, the more subtle the etiologic factors or events, the greater the sample size that is necessary to demonstrate the event.

Begin with a pilot study with simple, clearly stated objectives and a small, compatible team. Costs can be kept down by determining zygosity on clinical grounds. "Were you alike as two peas in a pod as children?" has over 95% accuracy in the United States in classifying twins.

Avoid selection bias of twin pairs so far as possible. Random selection from a large, heterogeneous patient population is ideal but seldom possible. Ascertainment from multiple sources is preferable to a single source.

Define and adhere strictly to criteria for diagnosis, whether on the clinical, or clinical and laboratory level. Expect a significant "diagnosis uncertain" group—and cherish them. They may well represent discrete subsets of the syndrome in question. Even among those fulfilling the diagnostic criteria look for patient groups that seem distinct, whether because of clinical findings, course, or laboratory results. Heterogeneity is the rule rather than the exception in complex syndromes.

Do not overinterpret from seemingly discordant twin groups where many are still within the age at risk. If at all possible, attempt to uncover subclinical cases by the most sensitive evaluation and long-term follow up, including autopsy.

Finally, don't be discouraged from considering a twin study simply because few twins have been reported. The Parkinson study revealed dramatically that the twins are there if sufficient patients are there. Just get out and find them!

REFERENCES

Currier, R. D., & Eldridge, R. Possible risk factors in multiple sclerosis as found in a national twin study. *Transactions of the American Neurological Association,* 1981, *105,* 304–305.

Currier, R. D., & Eldridge, R. Events influencing risks for MS. *Archives of Neurology,* 1982, 140–144.

Duvoisin, R. C., Gearing, F. R., Schweiger, M. D. *et al.* A family study of parkinsonism. In A. Barbeau & J. R. Brunette, (Eds.), *Progress in neurogenetics.* Amsterdam: Excerpta Medica, 1969.

Duvoisin, R. C., Eldridge, R., Williams, A., Nutt, J., & Calne, D. Twin study of Parkinson disease. *Neurology,* 1981, *31,* 77–80.

Eldridge, R., McFarland, H., Sever, J., Sadowsky, D., & Krebs, H. Familial multiple sclerosis: Clinical, histocompatibility, and viral serological studies. *Annals of Neurology,* 1978, *3,* 72–80.

Eldridge, R., McFarlin, D., & McFarland, H. *The NIH twin study in multiple sclerosis.* Unpublished Manuscript, in press, 1983.

Georgi, W. Multiple Sklerose. Pathologisch-anatomischa Refunde Multipler Sklerose bei klinisch nich diagnostizierten Krankheiten. *Schweigzerische Medizinische Wochenschrift,* 1961, *91,* 605.

Jenson, A. R. The heritability of intelligence. *Engineering and Science,* 1970, *6,* 1–206.

Klawans, H. L. Hemi-parkinson as a late complication of hemiatrophy: A new syndrome. *Neurology,* 1981, *31,* 605–608.

Kondo, K., Kurland, L. T., & Schull, W. J. Parkinson's disease, genetic analysis and evidence of a multifactorial etiology. *Mayo Clinic Proceedings,* 1973, *48,* 465–475.

Leske, M. C. Prevalence estimates of communicative disorders in the U.S. Speech disorders. *American Speech Hearing Association,* 1981, *23,* 217–225.

McFarlin, D., & Madden, D. *Survey of serum and CSF antibody between affected and unaffected MS twins.* Unpublished Manuscript, 1983.

Nance, W. E. A note on assortative mating and maternal effects. In *Genetic analysis of common diseases: Applications to predictive factors in coronary diseases.* New York: Alan R. Liss, 1979.

Rotter, J. I., & Rimoin, D. L. Heterogeneity in diabetes mellitus—update, 1978. Evidence for further genetic heterogeneity within juvenile-onset-insulin-dependent diabetes mellitus. *Diabetes,* 1978, *27,* 599–605.

Rotter, J. I. Genetic approaches to ulcer heterogeneity. In J. I. Rotter, J. M. Samloff, & D. L. Rimoin (Eds.), *The genetics and heterogeneity of common gastrointestinal disorders. New York:* Academic Press, *1980,* 111–128.

Schumacher, G. G., Beebe, G., Kibler, R. F. *et al.* Problems of experimental trials of therapy in multiple sclerosis. *Annals of New York Academy of Science,* 1965, *122,* 552–568.

Ward, C. D., Duvoisin, R. C., Ice, S. E., Nutt, J. D., Eldridge, R., & Calne, D. B. Parkinson disease in 65 pairs of twins and in a set of quadruplets. *Neurology* 1983, *33,* 815–824.

Williams, A., Eldridge, R., McFarland, H., Houff, S., Krebs, H., & McFarlin, D. Multiple sclerosis in twins. *Neurology,* 1980, *30,* 1139–1147.

8

Adoption Designs for the Study of Complex Behavioral Characters[1]

J. C. DeFRIES
ROBERT PLOMIN

INTRODUCTION

Many speech and language disorders, such as stuttering and reading disability, are characterized by familial transmission (e.g., Kidd, Heimbuch, & Records, 1981; DeFries & Decker, 1982). However, family studies cannot definitively determine whether such familiality is genetic or environmental in origin because nonadoptive family members share both heredity and common-family environmental influences. Although the demonstration of familial transmission is important (it is the sine qua non for genetic influence), adoption studies provide more convincing evidence for the inheritance of complex characters. Cavalli-Sforza (1975) has gone so far as to state that

> There is no way to distinguish between cultural and biological transmission unless one can study adoptions and test the similarity with *both* biological *and* adoptive relatives. . . . In the absence of adoption studies there is no hope of distinguishing rigorously whether standard measurements of inheritance, that is similarities between relatives (of any kind), are due to genetic determination of the trait differences, or to sociocultural inheritance (more generally, phenotypic transmission), or to a mixture of the two [p. 134].

In this chapter we shall outline how data from adoption studies can be used to test hypotheses of genetic influence, shared environmental influence, and

[1]The preparation of this chapter was supported in part by grants from the National Institute of Child Health and Human Development (HD-10333) and the National Science Foundation (BNS-7826204). We thank Rebecca G. Miles for expert editorial assistance.

121

GENETIC ASPECTS OF
SPEECH AND LANGUAGE DISORDERS

genotype–environment interactions and correlation. In addition, results from selected adoption studies will be reviewed and possible adoption designs for the study of speech and language disorders will be proposed.

ADOPTION MODELS

Parent–Offspring Resemblance

A path diagram depicting familial transmission of a character in a non-adoptive family is shown in Figure 8.1. The capital letter P symbolizes a parent's observed phenotypic value (e.g., a test score), G is a corresponding additive genetic value (Falconer, 1960), E_c and E_w are common-family and within-family environmental deviations, and the letters with the subscript o refer to these values and deviations for an offspring. It should be noted that E_c is due to environmental influences that cause members of a family to resemble one another, whereas E_w is due to environmental factors that are unique to each individual.

Figure 8.1 illustrates the point made earlier that parent–offspring resemblance in nonadoptive families is a function of both genetic and common-family environmental influences. More importantly, however, such models quantify the relative contributions of G and E_c to phenotypic resemblance. From path coefficient theory (Li, 1975), it can be shown that the parent–child correlation (r_{PP_o}) may be partitioned as follows:

$$r_{PP_o} = h^2 P_G + e_c^2, \tag{1}$$

where h^2 is narrow-sense heritability, P_G is a genetic path coefficient that equals .5 when mating is at random, and e_c^2 is common-family environmentality (see Plomin, DeFries, & McClearn, 1980).

A comparable diagram illustrating biological parent–adopted child and adoptive parent–adopted child resemblance is presented in Figure 8.2, where it

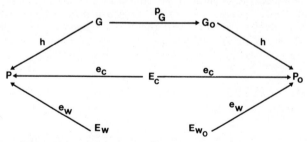

FIGURE 8.1. Path diagram of parent–child correlation in a control family. (From J. C. DeFries, R. Plomin, S. G. Vandenberg, & A. R. Kuse, "Parent–offspring resemblance for cognitive abilities in the Colorado Adoption Project: Biological, adoptive, and control parents and one-year-old children," *Intelligence*, 1981, 5, 245–277. Copyright 1981 by Ablex Publishing Corporation. Reprinted by permission.)

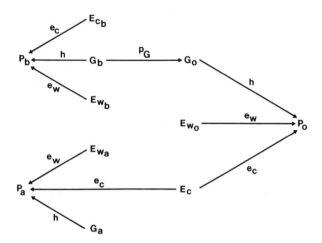

FIGURE 8.2. Path diagram of biological parent–adopted child and adoptive parent–adopted child correlations. (From J. C. DeFries, R. Plomin, S. G. Vandenberg, & A. R. Kuse, "Parent–offspring resemblance for cognitive abilities in the Colorado Adoption Project: Biological, adoptive, and control parents and one-year-old children," *Intelligence*, 1981, 5, 245–277. Copyright 1981 by Ablex Publishing Corporation. Reprinted by permission.)

is assumed that the adopted children were separated from their biological parents shortly after birth. From this figure it can be seen that such adopted children share genes with their biological parents, but only common-family environmental influences with their adoptive parents. In the absence of selective placement, the expected correlations between adopted children and their biological and adoptive parents, respectively, are as follows:

$$r_{P_b P_o} = h^2 p_G \tag{2}$$

and

$$r_{P_a P_o} = e_c^2. \tag{3}$$

By comparing Equation (1) with Equations (2) and (3), it becomes apparent how data from adoption studies can be used to partition familial resemblance in nonadoptive familes into genetic and environmental parts, that is,

$$r_{PP_o} = r_{P_b P_o} + r_{P_a P_o}. \tag{4}$$

From these equations it can also be seen that an estimate of genetic influence can be obtained even when no data are available from biological parents, namely:

$$r_{PP_o} - r_{P_a P_o} = h^2 p_G. \tag{5}$$

When the character under study is continuously distributed, expected correlations between family members are equated to observed correlations in order to estimate the various genetic and environmental parameters. However, when the character is dichotomous (e.g, stutterer versus normal), prevalence rates for the disorder in the relatives of affected individuals are compared to those in relatives of normals (see Plomin *et al.,* 1980). Two general designs are employed. In the adoptees' study method (see Figure 8.3), adoptees are ascertained through affected or normal biological parents. Therefore, an estimate of the importance of genetic influence is provided by a comparison of the prevalence in adoptees with an affected parent to that in those whose parents are unaffected. In contrast, with the adoptees' family method (see Figure 8.4) families are ascertained through affected and normal adoptees. With this method, prevalence rates in the biological parents of index cases (affected adoptees) are compared to those in their adoptive parents and to those in the biological and adoptive parents of controls. Examples of studies that have employed each of these methods will be described in a later section.

Sibling Resemblance

Sibling resemblance in nonadoptive families is depicted in Figure 8.5. Sibling resemblance in such families, of course, is also due both to genetic and common-family environmental influences:

$$\text{nonadoptive } r_{P_{O_1}P_{O_2}} = h^2 r_{G_O} + e_c^2, \tag{6}$$

where $r_{G_O} = .5$ when mating is at random. In contrast, in the absence of selective placement, adoptive sibling resemblance is due only to common-family environmental influence, that is:

$$\text{adoptive } r_{P_{O_1}P_{O_2}} = e_c^2. \tag{7}$$

Consequently, a comparison of sibling resemblance in adoptive and nonadop-

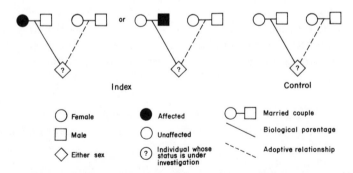

Index   Control

◯ Female	● Affected	◯⊸☐ Married couple
☐ Male	◯ Unaffected	╲ Biological parentage
◇ Either sex	⦾ Individual whose status is under investigation	---- Adoptive relationship

FIGURE 8.3. Pedigrees illustrating the adoptees' study method. (After R. Plomin, J. C. DeFries, & G. E. McClearn, "Behavioral genetics: A primer," San Francisco: Freeman, 1980, p. 344. Copyright 1980 by W. H. Freeman and Company. Reprinted by permission.)

FIGURE 8.4. Pedigrees illustrating the adoptees' family method. (After R. Plomin, J. C.
DeFries, & G. E. McClearn, "Behavioral genetics: A primer," San Francisco: Freeman,
1980, p. 344. Copyright 1980 by W. H. Freeman and Company. Reprinted by
permission.)

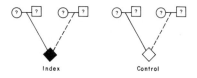

tive families can also be used to provide an estimate of the importance of genetic influence:

$$\text{nonadoptive } r_{P_{O_1}P_{O_2}} - \text{adoptive } r_{P_{O_1}P_{O_2}} = h^2 r_{G_O}. \qquad (8)$$

Although the same symbols have been employed for sibling and parent–offspring resemblance, it should be noted that e_c^2 estimated from sibling data may exceed that estimated from parent–child data. Siblings are more contemporaneous and, thus, are more likely to share life experiences. It should also be noted that E_c refers only to those environmental factors that are shared by family members and that cause their phenotypic resemblance. There may be other important environmental influences that are unique to each individual. As discussed in the following section, the importance of such specific environmental factors may be assessed independently of heredity in adoptive families.

Selective Placement

The highly simplified path models described in the preceding sections were included primarily for didactic purposes. In the real world of human genetics (especially human behavioral genetics), complications often arise. One complication that must be considered in a discussion of adoption studies is that of selective placement, that is, the nonrandom placement of adopted children in adoptive families.

A condensed model that depicts parent–offspring phenotypic re-

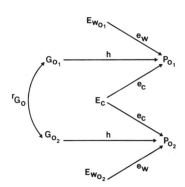

FIGURE 8.5. Path diagram of sibling correlation in a
control family.

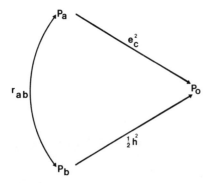

FIGURE 8.6. Path diagram of parent–child resemblance when there is a correlation between adoptive parent (P_a) and biological parent (P_b) due to selective placement. (From J. C. DeFries, R. Plomin, S. G. Vandenberg, & A. R. Kuse, "Parent–offspring resemblance for cognitive abilities in the Colorado Adoption Project: Biological, adoptive, and control parents and one-year-old children," *Intelligence*, 1981, *5*, 245–277. Copyright 1981 by Ablex Publishing Corporation. Reprinted by permission.)

semblance in the presence of selective placement is shown in Figure 8.6. From this figure it can be seen that both biological parent–adopted child and adoptive parent–adopted child correlations are functions of the correlation between the adoptive and biological parents (r_{ab}), that is,

$$r_{P_bP_o} = \tfrac{1}{2}h^2 + r_{ab}e_c^2 \tag{9}$$

and

$$r_{P_aP_o} = e_c^2 + \tfrac{1}{2}r_{ab}h^2. \tag{10}$$

Thus, in the presence of positive selective placement, biological parent–adopted child correlations can yield overestimates of the importance of genetic influence, and adoptive parent–adopted child correlations can result in overestimates of common-family environmental influence. As a consequence, it is imperative that selective placement be assessed in an adoption study in order to determine whether it is necessary to control its influence statistically.

Assortative Mating

Another complication that can arise in adoption studies is that due to assortative mating. Although less well recognized as a problem than selective placement, it can also result in biased estimates of genetic and environmental influences. Data from biological fathers are seldom obtained in an adoption study. Therefore, estimates of the importance of genetic influence are usually based solely upon biological mother–adopted child resemblance. However, it is well known that parent–child correlations are a function of the mate correlation. To illustrate this principle, a path diagram depicting biological parent–adopted child resemblance in the presence of phenotypic assortative mating is presented in Figure 8.7. From this figure it can be seen that the expected biological mother–adopted child correlation is a function of the mate correlation (t), as follows:

$$r_{P_{bm}P_o} = \tfrac{1}{2}h^2(1 + t). \tag{11}$$

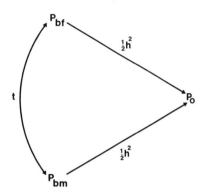

FIGURE 8.7. Path diagram of biological parent–adopted child resemblance when there is a correlation between biological parents (t). (From J. C. DeFries, R. Plomin, S. G. Vandenberg, & A. R. Kuse, "Parent–offspring resemblance for cognitive abilities in the Colorado Adoption Project: Biological, adoptive, and control parents and one-year-old children," *Intelligence*, 1981, 5, 245–277. Copyright 1981 by Ablex Publishing Corporation. Reprinted by permission.)

As mate correlations for unwed parents may differ from those for adoptive or nonadoptive couples, it is important to attempt to obtain at least some information from biological fathers in an adoption study.

A similar problem exists for adoptive family correlations. For example, from Figure 8.8 it can be seen that the expected adoptive mother–adopted child correlation is as follows:

$$r_{P_{am}P_o} = e^2_{cm} + e^2_{cf} t, \tag{12}$$

where e^2_{cm} and e^2_{cf} are proportions of variance due to maternal and paternal environmental influences, respectively. Therefore, measures of assortative mating should be obtained for biological parents, adoptive parents, and nonadoptive parents if at all possible in an adoption study.

Specific Environmental Influences

Measures of the home environment often correlate with children's behavior. For example, dozens of studies—many using the Home Observation for

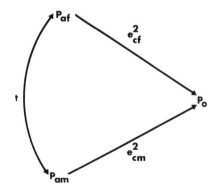

FIGURE 8.8. Path diagram of adoptive parent–adopted child resemblance when there is a correlation between adoptive parents (t). (From J. C. DeFries, R. Plomin, S. G. Vandenberg, & A. R. Kuse, "Parent–offspring resemblance for cognitive abilities in the Colorado Adoption Project: Biological, adoptive, and control parents and one-year-old children," *Intelligence*, 1981, 5, 245–277. Copyright 1981 by Ablex Publishing Corporation. Reprinted by permission.)

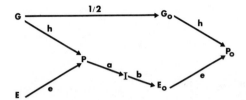

FIGURE 8.9. Path diagram of correlation between an environmental index (I) and an offspring phenotype (P_o) in a control family.

Measurement of the Environment (HOME) instrument of Caldwell and Bradley (1978)—have reported that aspects of the home environment are related to infant cognitive development in nonadoptive families. However, as shown in Figure 8.9, such a relationship may be due at least in part to hereditary influences:

$$r_{IP_o} = be + \tfrac{1}{2}h^2a, \tag{13}$$

where I is an index of environmental influence. The usual way of thinking about the relationship between I and P_o is to view it as being mediated entirely environmentally (i.e., by way of b and e). However, the environmental index may be a function of the parental phenotype (path a). For example, in an economically heterogeneous study of 41 families, Campbell (1979) obtained correlations exceeding .70 between mothers' IQ and HOME total scores. The HOME scores also correlated .69 with 4-year-old Stanford-Binet IQ scores. Thus, the HOME correlates as much with parental IQ as it does with children's IQ. A recent study using a different home environment measure obtained similar results (Longstreth, Davis, Canter, Flint, Owen, Rickert, & Taylor, 1981). Because parental phenotype is correlated with offspring phenotype due to genetic factors, the possibility of a genetic confound in such ostensibly environmental relationships looms large.

In contrast, environmental assessments embedded in an adoption study facilitate strong tests of the importance of specific environmental influences that are not confounded by heredity. From the path diagram shown in Figure 8.10, it can be seen that (in the absence of selective placement) the correlation between I and P_o in adoptive families provides a direct measure of the environ-

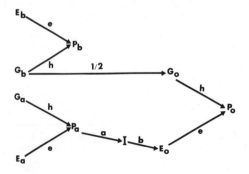

FIGURE 8.10. Path diagram of correlation between an environmental index (I) and an offspring phenotype (P_o) in an adoptive family.

mental relationship. Parenthetically, it is interesting to note that the best evidence for environmental influence may ultimately result from application of behavioral genetic designs.

GENOTYPE–ENVIRONMENT (*GE*) INTERACTION AND CORRELATION

As has been outlined, adoption studies facilitate estimates of the importance of the separate effects of heredity and environment. However, genes and environment do not operate in a vacuum and their effects are not always independent. A major advantage of adoption studies is that adoption data can be utilized to test for the presence of *GE* interactions and correlations.

Definitions

Genotype–Environment interaction refers to the differential response of different genotypes to environmental influences. For example, certain forms of therapy or remediation may work better for some children than others. In contrast, *GE* correlation is defined as the nonrandom exposure of different genotypes to different environments. In previous writings, we (Plomin, DeFries, & Loehlin, 1977) have distinguished three different types of *GE* correlation: passive, reactive, and active (see Table 8.1).

Passive *GE* correlation occurs when parents provide their children with both genes and an environment that are favorable (or unfavorable) for the development of a particular trait. A widely cited example is verbal ability, where parents who are highly verbal provide their children with both genes (to the extent that verbal ability is inherited) and an environment that is conducive to the development of verbal ability. This form of *GE* correlation is labeled *passive* because it occurs independently of the behavior of the recipient.

TABLE 8.1
Three Types of Genotype–Environment Correlation[a]

Type	Description	Pertinent environment
Passive	Children are given genotypes linked to their environments	Natural parents
Reactive	Children are reacted to on the basis of their genotype	Anybody
Active	Children seek an environment conducive to their genotype	Anything

[a]From R. Plomin, J. C. DeFries, & J. C. Loehlin, "Genotype–environment interaction and correlation in the analysis of human behavior," *Psychological Bulletin,* 1977, *84,* 309–322. Copyright 1977 by the American Psychological Association. Reprinted by permission.

TABLE 8.2
Illustrative Design for Testing Genotype-by-Environment Interaction

Genotype	Environment	
	Low	High
Low	P_{11}	P_{12}
High	P_{21}	P_{22}

In contrast, reactive *GE* correlation occurs when people react differently to persons of different genotypes. Reactive *GE* correlation is not limited to environments provided by relatives and is dependent upon the behavior of the recipient. Teachers, for example, may attempt to maximize the performance of children of different abilities by utilizing different strategies, thereby contributing to reactive *GE* correlation. In fact, the whole concept of individualized instruction could foster a nonrandom association of genotypes and environments.

Finally, active *GE* correlation is due to the voluntary selection of different environments by individuals of different genotypes. Highly intelligent children, for example, may seek situations, peers, games, books, etc., that foster their further intellectual development.

Tests of *GE* Interaction and Correlation

Although *GE* interactions may be of considerable importance for complex human behavioral characters, very few attempts have been made to test for their presence. One reason for this is the lack of appropriate tests. We have proposed one test for *GE* interaction that utilizes adoption data (Plomin *et al.*, 1977). The test is analogous to that used in animal studies where different strains are reared in different environments. However, rather than using strains as an independent variable, measures obtained from the biological parents are used as an index of the adopted child's genotype. Aspects of the adoptive home are also assessed. For didactic purposes, we suggested that scores of the biological parents and measures of the environment be dichotomized (high versus low). Scores for the adopted children are then cross-tabulated (see Table 8.2) and subjected to a 2 × 2 analysis of variance from which the significance of both main effects (genetic and environmental) and their interaction can be ascertained. For a more exact significance test, we recommend that continuous data be subjected to hierarchical multiple regression analysis (Cohen & Cohen, 1975).

Tests for the presence of *GE* correlation differ for the three types described above. As biological parents transmit genes but not environmental influences, passive *GE* correlation cannot occur for adopted children in the absence of selective placement. Phenotypic variance in a population, of course, contains components due to G, E, $G \times E$, and $2CovGE$. Therefore, the phenotypic variance in a population of adopted children should be less than that in a population of nonadopted children if passive GE correlation is important (and positive). Tests of active and reactive GE correlation require assessments of various aspects of the adopted child's environment (e.g., child-rearing practices of the adoptive parents) which may be correlated with measures of the biological parents.

To date, little effort has been expended to search for GE interactions or correlations in human populations. Nevertheless, it is our conviction that the use of adoption data to screen for possible GE interactions and correlations is an unusually promising approach for understanding the etiology of individual differences.

EXAMPLES OF ADOPTION STUDIES

Adoption studies of schizophrenia, criminality, alcoholism, hyperactivity, and mental ability have been reviewed in detail (e.g., DeFries & Plomin, 1978). Because of space limitations, only three of these studies will be described here.

Colorado Adoption Project (CAP)

Data in the ongoing CAP (DeFries, Plomin, Vandenberg, & Kuse, 1981) are obtained on biological (unwed) parents who relinquish their children for adoption, on adoptive parents who adopt these children, on nonadoptive parents rearing their own children (controls), and on both the adopted and control children. The adults are administered a 3-hour battery of behavioral tests related to specific cognitive abilities and personality. In addition, extensive questionnaire data pertaining to demographic characteristics, commonly used drugs, common behavior problems (e.g., headaches, phobias, neuroses), interests and talents, handedness, food preferences, speech problems, and height and weight are obtained. Children are currently being tested yearly between 1 and 4 years of age and additional testing is planned at 7, 11, and 16 years. Behavioral assessments for the children include standard objective tests of cognitive abilities, interview data provided by parents, videotape recordings of parental and child behavior, and environmental assessments. The CAP is unique in a number of respects: It is longitudinal in design; the sample is large (our goal is to include a total of 300 adoptive and 300 control families in the study); the approach is multivariate; the environment provided in the homes is measured by standardized instruments; when possible, biological fathers are tested as well as biological mothers; and a control sample of nonadoptive families is matched to the adoptive families for age, family structure, and socioeconomic status.

Although the CAP has been in progress for over 5 years, only preliminary analyses of the partial data set have been reported (DeFries *et al.*, 1981). Data

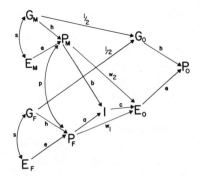

FIGURE 8.11. Path diagram of correlations between parents (P_M, P_F), a child (P_o), and an environmental index (I) in Colorado Adoption Project control families.

were summarized for 359 biological parents, 261 adoptive parents, 154 control parents, and 119 adopted and 79 control 1-year-old children. Analyses of the adult data indicated that biological, adoptive, and control parents are highly similar with regard to various demographic variables, test reliabilities, cognitive test score variances and factor structure, and mate correlations. Moreover, selective placement was found to be nonsignificant. This latter was expected as the agencies participating in the study do not consciously match biological and adoptive parents on any systematic basis and would have little opportunity to do so even if they tried. A detailed description of the demographic characteristics of the sample, its ascertainment, and the tests and measurements employed has also been reported (see DeFries *et al.*, 1981).

Path diagrams depicting relationships among the cognitive variables for members of control and adoptive families in the CAP are presented in Figures 8.11 and 8.12. An environmental index (I) is assumed to be a function of the adoptive and control parental phenotypes and causally related to the child's environment (E_o). Independent contributions of parental phenotype not mediated by the index are also indicated (w_1 and w_2). Correlations due to selective placement (x_1, x_2, x_3, x_4), assortative mating (p and q), and GE correlation (s) are also included. It should be emphasized that these figures are only to be

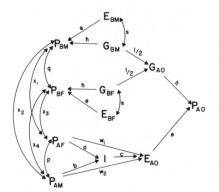

FIGURE 8.12. Path diagram of correlations between biological parents (P_{BM}, P_{BF}) and an adopted child (P_{AO}) and between adoptive parents (P_{AF}, P_{AM}) and an adopted child (P_{AO}) in the Colorado Adoption Project.

TABLE 8.3
Maximum Likelihood Parameter Estimates (S.E.) from CAP Cognitive Data
on Biological, Adoptive, and Control Parents and Their One-Year-Old Children

	Full model		Partial model
h	.42	(.14)	.51 (.10)
s	−.001	(.10)	—
w_1	.14	(.07)	—
w_2	.04	(.08)	—
p	.18	(.06)	.19 (.07)
q	.32	(.33)	.32 (.33)
x_1	.06	(.08)	—
x_2	−.04	(.10)	—
x_3	.12	(.16)	—
x_4	.28	(.18)	—
a	.09	(.07)	—
b	.01	(.07)	—
c	.17	(.08)	.20 (.08)
	$\chi^2_{50} = 55.94$		$\chi^2_{58} = 64.58$

regarded as being of heuristic value at this stage of analysis and are by no
means either final or definitive.

Utilizing these path models, expected covariances among the variables
were derived and then equated to observed covariances to solve for the various
parameters (DeFries, Plomin, & Fulker, 1980). In order to use all available data
most efficiently, a maximum likelihood model fitting procedure developed by
Fulker (1978) was employed. A set of five independent covariance matrices
based upon complete and nonoverlapping subsets of the data (first principal
component score for adults, Bayley mental scores for 1-year-old children, and
Caldwell's HOME responsivity scale as an environmental index) was equated to
the expected covariances using an optimization error analysis routine made
available by CERN (1977).

Results of this analysis are summarized in Table 8.3. From this table it may
be seen that h is highly significant, suggesting the presence of a genetic relationship between general cognitive ability of parents and Bayley mental scores
of their 1-year-old children. The path c from the index to the child's environmental deviation is also significant, indicating a direct influence of environmental factors measured by Caldwell's HOME responsivity scale. It is interesting to
note, however, that parental general cognitive ability is not related to the index in
our study, that is, paths a and b are nonsignificant. Moreover, parental general
cognitive ability does not relate to the child's environment independently of the
index (w_1 and w_2 are not significant). Although assortative mating for adoptive
and control couples is significant, it is relatively modest in size ($p = .18$). Finally,
selective placement (x_1, x_2, x_3, x_4) and GE correlation (s) are not significant in
this study.

These preliminary analyses of CAP data illustrate the utility of the maximum likelihood model fitting appraoch. The model is made explicit by the path diagrams, and all data and parameters are analyzed simultaneously. Another major advantage of this approach is that it facilitates tests of alternative models. For example, as shown in Table 8.3, a much simpler model fits the data almost as well as the full model.

Alternative analyses of CAP data are currently in progress. For example, a longitudinal analysis is being conducted in which scores of children at more than one age are analyzed simultaneously. In addition, different models of environmental transmission and multivariate extensions are under investigation.

Schizophrenia

In the CAP, ascertainment of subjects was through the biological parents of adoptees. In some of the classical adoption studies of psychopathology (e.g., Heston, 1966; Rosenthal, Wender, Kety, Schulsinger, Welner, & Ostergaard, 1968), the adoptees' study method was also used, that is, ascertainment of subjects at risk for psychopathology was through biological parents of adopted children. For example, in Heston's study, an experimental group of 47 young adults born to schizophrenic mothers, but permanently separated from them during the first month of life and subsequently reared in foster or adoptive homes, was compared to 50 controls (adoptees or foster children born to mothers with no record of psychiatric disturbance). Heston assessed the behavior of these adoptees by various means, including psychiatric interviews and reviews of school, police, medical, and Veterans Administration records. As can be seen from Table 8.4, there are a number of indications of increased psychopathology among the experimental subjects. Moreover, there were five diagnosed cases of schizophrenia among the experimental group versus none in the control group, a result highly consistent with a hypothesis of genetic influence.

A similar conclusion based upon results of an adoption study employing the adoptees' family method was reached by Kety, Rosenthal, Wender, Schulsinger, and Jacobsen (1975) several years later. Kety et al. (1975) utilized the "Folkeregister" in Copenhagen, Denmark, to locate approximately 5500 individuals who had been adopted between 1924 and 1947. Among these adoptees, hospital records indicated that 33 could be diagnosed as falling within the hard-core schizophrenic spectrum. These index adoptees were matched to controls (adoptees with no psychiatric history) for sex, age, age at placement in the adoptive home, and socioeconomic status of the adoptive family. The Folkeregister was then searched for the names of biological and adoptive relatives of both groups of adoptees. Almost all of the biological and adoptive parents and a large number of biological half-siblings were found. Approximately 90% of these relatives were interviewed and psychiatric diagnoses were obtained. The prevalence of schizophrenia (hard-core schizophrenic spectrum)

TABLE 8.4
**Results of Heston's Study of Persons Born to Schizophrenic Mothers and Reared in Adoptive
or Foster Homes, and of Controls Born to Normal Parents and Similarly Reared[a]**

Item	Control	Experimental	Exact probability (Fisher's test)
Number of subjects	50	47	
Number of males	33	30	
Age, mean	36.3	35.8	
MHSRS means[b]	80.1	65.2	.0006
Number with schizophrenia	0	5	.024
Number with antisocial personalities	2	9	.017
Number with neurotic personality disorder	7	13	.052
Number spending more than 1 year in penal or psychiatric institution	2	11	.006
Number serving in armed forces	17	21	
Number discharged from armed forces on psychiatric or behavioral grounds	1	8	.021
Social group, first home, mean	4.2	4.5	
Social group, present, mean	4.7	5.4	
Years in school, mean	12.4	11.6	
Number of divorces, total	7	6	
Number never married, > 30 years of age	4	9	

[a]From L. L. Heston, "The genetics of schizophrenic and schizoid disease," *Science,* 1970, *167,* 249–256. Copyright 1970 by the American Association for the Advancement of Science. Reprinted by permission.
[b]The MHSRS is a global rating of psychopathology moving from 0 to 100 with decreasing psychopathology. Total group mean, 72.8; S.D., 18.4.

found in the biological and adoptive relatives of the schizophrenic and non-schizophrenic adoptees is summarized in Table 8.5. These data are highly consistent with previous results indicating a significant genetic influence. Moreover, the finding that the prevalence among paternal half-siblings (same father, different mothers) is similar to that for maternal half-sibs suggests that both prenatal and early postnatal environmental factors are not important etiological determinants of familial transmission of schizophrenia.

POSSIBLE ADOPTION DESIGNS FOR THE STUDY OF SPEECH AND LANGUAGE DISORDERS

Adoption studies of speech and language disorders could employ either the adoptees' study method or the adoptees' family method. In fact, a prospective study of stuttering employing the former method is currently in progress. As part of the CAP, personal and family history data pertaining to speech problems

TABLE 8.5
Hard-Core Schizophrenic Spectrum (Based on Psychiatric Interviews) in Biological and Adoptive Relatives of Schizophrenic and Nonschizophrenic Adoptees[a]

	Nonschizophrenic adoptees	Schizophrenic adoptees
First-degree biological relatives	4% (3/68)	12% (8/68)
Adoptive parents and siblings	4% (4/90)	3% (2/73)
Biological half-siblings (total sample)	3% (3/104)	16% (16/101)
Biological half-siblings (paternal only)	3% (2/64)	18% (11/61)

[a]From S. S. Kety, D. Rosenthal, P. H. Wender, F. Schulsinger, and B. Jacobsen, "Mental illness in the biological and adoptive families of adopted individuals who have become schizophrenic: A preliminary report based on psychiatric interviews," *Genetic Research in Psychiatry* (edited by R. R. Fieve, D. Rosenthal, and H. Brill), Baltimore: Johns Hopkins University Press, 1975, pp. 147–166. Copyright 1975 by Johns Hopkins University Press. Reprinted by permission.

are being collected for biological, adoptive, and control parents in collaboration with Dr. Kenneth K. Kidd. As expected, of the 1044 CAP adults tested to date, only 32 have indicated a personal history of stuttering or stammering (4 biological fathers, 10 biological mothers, 5 adoptive fathers, 2 adoptive mothers, 6 control fathers, and 5 control mothers). Thus, although we will be able to ascertain the prevalence of speech and language problems in children of biological and adoptive parents with the disorder, the number of children at risk in the CAP will be rather small. On the other hand, if the character could be quantified (i.e., if the disorder could be regarded as being the extreme end of a continuous distribution), and if the etiology of individual differences within the normal range is similar to that at the extremes, then a prospective adoption study of speech and language disorders in an unselected population, such as the CAP sample, could be very informative.

A more targeted study of adoptees at risk could be accomplished by studying only children whose biological or adoptive parents manifest the problem. However, given the low frequency of such disorders and the drastic decline in the number of adoptive placements that has occurred during the last decade, it would be difficult to obtain an adequate sample.

On the other hand, a retrospective study employing the adoptees' family method is entirely feasible. With the cooperation of several adoption agencies, questionnaires pertaining to speech and language problems of the adoptee could be mailed to families in which an adopted child has been placed during the previous 10–15 years. More extensive questionnaires could be mailed to families of affected adoptees, or interviews could be arranged. As shown in Figure 8.13, affected children in nonadoptive families could be matched to the adoptees and the prevalence of disorders in their families could be ascertained. A comparison of the prevalence rates in adoptive family members of affected adoptees to those in nonadoptive family members of affected control children would provide a test of the importance of genetic influence. Tests of common-

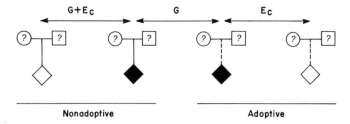

Nonadoptive   Adoptive

FIGURE 8.13. Pedigrees illustrating the design of a possible adoption study of speech and language disorders. As explained in the text, the symbols G and E_c refer to information gleaned from the comparison of the pedigrees connected by arrows. For example, evidence of genetic influence (G) is obtained by comparing the prevalence of a disorder in parents of nonadoptive probands to the prevalence in adoptive parents of adopted probands.

family environmental influence could be accomplished if prevalence rates were also obtained for family members of unaffected matched controls and/or adoptees.

It seems to us that such a study could yield significant results. For example, one of the agencies that has collaborated with us placed approximately 1000 children during the last decade. Assuming cooperation by four such agencies, a prevalence rate of 3% for a disorder of interest, and a 50% rate of participation, 60 affected adoptees would be identified. Given a 20% risk to first-degree relatives in nonadoptive families and only a 3% risk in adoptive families, a highly significant difference should be obtained (especially when the data are pooled across mothers, fathers, and siblings). Moreover, it would not be necessary to confine the study to a single disorder. Several different speech and language disorders could be studied simultaneously. By analyzing the resulting data set both isomorphically (character X in both parents and children) and hetero-morphically (character X in parents and character Y in offspring), genetic and environmental correlates between the characters could also be investigated.

Progressive adoption agencies with which we have collaborated in Colorado recognize the importance of research and have been very responsive to requests for cooperation as long as the projects are conducted in a discrete and nonintrusive manner. Thus, it is our opinion that definitive evidence regarding the etiology of speech and language disorders could be obtained from a retrospective adoption study and that such a study should be considered for possible implementation.

REFERENCES

Caldwell, B. M., & Bradley, R. H. *Home observation for measurement of the environment.* Little Rock: University of Arkansas, 1978.

Campbell, F. *How shall the IQ be measured?* Paper presented at the biennial meeting of the Society for Research in Child Development, San Francisco, 1979.

Cavalli-Sforza, L. L. Quantitative genetic perspectives. In K. W. Schaie, V. E. Anderson, G. E.

McClearn, & J. Money (Eds.), *Developmental human behavior genetics.* Lexington, Mass.: D. C. Heath, 1975.

CERN Computer Centre. *MINUIT: A system for function minimization and analysis of parameter errors and correlations.* Geneva: CERN, 1977.

Cohen, J., & Cohen, P. *Applied multiple regression/correlation analysis for the behavioral sciences.* Hillsdale, N.J.: Lawrence Erlbaum, 1975.

DeFries, J. C., & Decker, S. N. Genetic aspects of reading disability: A family study. In R. N. Malatesha & P. G. Aaron (Eds.), *Reading disorders: Varieties and treatments.* New York: Academic Press, 1982.

DeFries, J. C., & Plomin, R. Behavioral genetics. *Annual Review of Psychology,* 1978, *29,* 473–515.

DeFries, J. C., Plomin, R., & Fulker, D. W. Unpublished, 1980.

DeFries, J. C., Plomin, R., Vandenberg, S. G., & Kuse, A. R. Parent–offspring resemblance for cognitive abilities in the Colorado Adoption Project: Biological, adoptive, and control parents and one-year-old children. *Intelligence,* 1981,*5,* 245–277.

Falconer, D. S. *Introduction to quantitative genetics.* New York: Ronald Press, 1960.

Fulker, D. W. Multivariate extensions of a biometrical model of twin data. In W. E. Nance (Ed.), *Twin research: Psychology and methodology.* New York: Alan R. Liss, 1978.

Heston, L. L. Psychiatric disorders in foster home reared children of schizophrenic mothers. *British Journal of Psychiatry,* 1966, *112,* 819–825.

Heston, L. L. The genetics of schizophrenic and schizoid disease. *Science,* 1970, *167,* 249–256.

Kety, S. S., Rosenthal, D., Wender, P. H., Schulsinger, F., & Jacobsen, B. Mental illness in the biological and adoptive families of adopted individuals who have become schizophrenic: A preliminary report based on psychiatric interviews. In R. R. Fieve, D. Rosenthal, & H. Brill (Eds.), *Genetic research in psychiatry.* Baltimore: Johns Hopkins University Press, 1975.

Kidd, K. K., Heimbuch, R. C., & Records, M. A. Vertical transmission of susceptibility to stuttering with sex-modified expression. *Proceedings of the National Academy of Sciences,* 1981, *78,* 606–610.

Li, C. C. *Path analysis: A primer.* Pacific Grove, Calif.: Boxwood Press, 1975.

Longstreth, L. E., Davis, B., Canter, L., Flint, D., Owen, J., Rickert, M., & Taylor, E. Separation of home intellectual environment and maternal IQ as determinants of child IQ. *Developmental Psychology,* 1981, *17,* 532–541.

Plomin, R., DeFries, J. C., & Loehlin, J. C. Genotype–environment interaction and correlation in the analysis of human behavior. *Psychological Bulletin,* 1977, *84,* 309–322.

Plomin, R., DeFries, J. C., & McClearn, G. E. *Behavioral genetics: A primer.* San Francisco: Freeman, 1980.

Rosenthal, D., Wender, P. H., Kety, S. S., Schulsinger, F., Welner, J., & Ostergaard, L. Schizophrenics' offspring reared in adoptive homes. In D. Rosenthal & S. S. Kety (Eds.), *The transmission of schizophrenia.* London: Pergamon Press, 1968.

9

Genetic Analysis of Family Pedigree Data: A Review of Methodology[1]

DAVID L. PAULS

INTRODUCTION

Speech and language disorders present many of the same problems to genetic researchers as do other complex disorders. The etiologies are either unknown or poorly understood, and the specific pathogenesis for each disorder is largely unknown. No clear single-locus etiology is evidenced either by a specific biochemical defect or by a Mendelian pattern in families. Attempts to understand these complex behaviors require advancement on several fronts: nosologic, physiological, and genetic. The purpose of this chapter is to review some genetic methodologies, their strengths and limitations, their prerequisites and/or assumptions, and the inferences that can be drawn from the results. These methods are potentially useful in determining whether genetic models can adequately explain the observed patterns in families. Therefore, I will review, very briefly, some genetic models suitable for speech and language disorders. First, some general comments regarding genetic models.

Genetic models for complex traits serve as hypotheses that relate genes and genotypes, their frequencies in the population, and other relevant variables to the phenotypes and the distributions of phenotypes within the population and within individual families. These models can aid in the design of data collection strategies that will optimize the amount of relevant information collected. Using a genetic model for analyzing specific traits can thus provide considerable insight into the biology of the disorder.

[1]This work was supported in part by National Institutes of Health grants NS 11786 and NS 16648.

All genetic models make several assumptions that are very likely to be violated by any biological system. Although the degree to which specific assumptions are violated and the effect on any outcome may be trivial, the effect may also be sufficient to invalidate an analysis, and researchers must always be aware that these assumptions are being made. The most common assumption made is that of a gaussian distribution. Whether that be the distribution of error or the distribution of genetic effects, it is nevertheless an assumed distribution which usually cannot be directly validated. In addition, most models that involve more than one factor also assume a simple additive interaction of those factors at some level. The existence of a normal distribution for phenotype does not constitute proof that underlying factors interact in a simple additive fashion. Another assumption frequently made is that there exists a parameter (or parameters) labeled penetrance. Penetrance is an abstraction and exists only as a probability over many individuals. The actual mechanism that determines whether a given person with a susceptible genotype does or does not manifest the trait may be unique to that individual. This does not invalidate the concept of penetrance but does limit its biologic interpretation.

Two related considerations must always be held as caveats in analyses of complex traits like speech and language disorders: the definition of the phenotype and genetic-etiologic heterogeneity. Since genetic models relate the underlying genetic mechanism to a specific set of phenotypes, a redefinition of that set of phenotypes may substantially alter the parameters of a model. As described in what follows, some genetic models allow for one definition of phenotype in the proband and a different, though related, definition in family members. In general, however, unless otherwise explicitly stated in a model, genetic models assume a single definition for the phenotype of a disorder. In addition, models being considered here also assume that the specific disorder in question has a single basic etiology and no allowance is made, except as an error term, for completely separate genetic–etiologic mechanisms leading to the same disorder.

Although one could consider models that permit two or more independent genetic etiologies for the disorder, that seems unlikely to be a profitable scheme. The course most frequently pursued is to strive for data sets in which the disorder is likely to be as homogeneous as possible. That can be achieved by (a) defining the phenotype as rigorously as possible, (b) controlling for possible relevant nongenetic variables, and (c) collecting data from a population as genetically homogeneous as possible.

One important factor in analyses using genetic models is deciding which parameters to fix at predetermined values and which parameters to estimate in the context of fitting the models. Some of the models may appear to have very few parameters only because some parameters are judged to be less important or to have known fixed values. In different analytic methods for the same model there may be different numbers of parameters. For example, though basically following the single-major-locus model, segregation analysis using GENPED

(Kaplan & Elston, 1976) has several parameters not included in other methods, such as the segregation probabilities. In some methods parameters are optional: sex-specific parameters may easily be incorporated into most models; the parameters for a variable age of onset can be included in a pedigree analysis or linkage analysis and estimated simultaneously with the other parameters. Unfortunately, when more parameters are estimated from a finite amount of data, all the parameter estimates will be less precise. Therefore, whenever possible, preliminary analyses should be done in the hope of reducing the number of parameters estimated with the analysis, either by fixing their values or by eliminating them altogether.

A final point that deserves emphasis is the importance of hypothesis testing. This can be seen from two different perspectives. First, general qualitative agreement of a data set with the predications of a hypothesis does not constitute a statistical test of that hypothesis. It may very well be that the data do not show the specific quantitative relationships predicted by the model even though the general trends agree. Alternatively, as popularized by Popper (1959), scientific understanding advances primarily by excluding hypotheses. This latter perspective is especially relevant in the case of genetic models, as frequently two or more quite different genetic models have given statistically acceptable fits to a given set of data. This seems to be a general phenomenon because apparently most common types of patterns within families can often be explained equally well by quite divergent hypotheses. Reasonable hypotheses appear to differ primarily, that is, to the greatest degree, in their predictions for very uncommon familial constellations (e.g., the risk of two normal parents having four affected children) (Kidd, 1979). Even very large data sets may be quite deficient in that specific information that is most discriminating among hypotheses. Hence, finding a hypothesis with which the data are compatible cannot be considered as strong support for that hypothesis. The hypothesis should serve only as a guide for further research designed to eventually elucidate the genetic and environmental factors, and their interactions, that are relevant to the etiology of the disorder.

SPECIFIC MODELS THAT MAY BE APPROPRIATE FOR SPEECH AND LANGUAGE DISORDERS

In what follows, several specific models and methodologies appropriate for each model will be discussed. Each of the models makes many simplifying assumptions and the methods appropriate for those models have many mathematical restrictions. However, they do provide ways of looking at family data and are useful first steps to understanding the biology of complex traits.

Multifactorial-Polygenic Model (MFP)

The assumptions that characterize the classical multifactorial-polygenic model are as follows: (a) A quantitative trait, P, may be partitioned as $P = A + E,$

where A denotes the transmitted factors that contribute to the expression of the trait and E denotes all other random environmental influences on the trait, with the covariance (A, E) equal to zero; (b) the multiple transmitted factors are of small, equal, and additive effect relative to the total phenotypic variance; and (c) the phenotypic distribution is assumed to be normal.

Unfortunately, speech and language disorders are not quantitative traits, so the preceding model is not directly applicable. Although there are gradations of severity with these disorders, there are definite categories of "affected" and "unaffected." The multifactorial model for qualitative traits was first described by Crittenden (1961) and Falconer (1965). They postulated an underlying liability scale which satisfies all of the preceding criteria. Liability is defined as the sum of all events both genetic and environmental that contribute to the expression of the trait. A threshold on the liability scale, presumably a reflection of some physiological phenomenon, divides the distribution into affected and unaffected individuals. Any individuals with a sufficient number of factors for the trait (whether genetic or environmental) will exceed the threshold and be classified as affected.

Utilizing the properties of the normal distribution, population incidence of the trait, and incidence in various classes of relatives, it is possible to estimate the heritability for any trait (Falconer, 1965), but a goodness-of-fit test is not possible. Other methodologies have been developed to utilize the actual pedigree structures to estimate parameters and to test the MFP model (Lange, Westlake, & Spence, 1976; Gladstien, Lange, & Spence, 1978). Unfortunately, pedigree data are not always available to test the model. Because this is so, Reich, James, and Morris (1972) have generalized the original model to include multiple thresholds. The multiple thresholds can correspond to different forms of the disorder, different frequencies between the sexes, or a combination of the two. This generalization allows the use of family prevalence data for both parameter estimation and a statistical goodness-of-fit test. The only requirement is that it be possible to divide the data on affected into at least two categories (e.g., levels of severity or different frequencies between the sexes) that differ in mean liability. This model (with only two thresholds) is completely defined by three parameters: (a) the population prevalence for the more common form of the disorder (or the more common sex), (b) the population prevalence of the less common form of the disorder (or less common sex), and (c) the correlation between relatives. If the values of these parameters are known, expected values can be calculated for all prevalences of one type of the disorder for relatives of probands of the other type. These expected values are then compared to those observed in the data.

The Single-Major-Locus (SML) or
Two-Allele Autosomal Locus (TAAL) Model

The simplest alternative to the multifactorial-polygenic model is one in which the genetic or transmitted component is attributable entirely to segregation at a single locus with two alternative alleles. Development of the general mathematical formulation of this model took place in the early 1970s (Morton, Yee, & Lew, 1971; Elston & Campbell, 1971; James, 1971; Elandt-Johnson, 1970). The model can be conceptualized in two different forms: a graphical representation on a liability scale (Cavalli-Sforza & Kidd, 1972) or a more strictly algebraic formulation in which genotypes are assigned penetrances (James, 1971). These two conceptualizations of the model can be mathematically equivalent under certain limiting assumptions. In the simplest algebraic formulation of the model, the four parameters are the frequency, q, for one of the alleles (e.g., a, the allele associated most strongly with the disorder) and three penetrances, f_0, f_1, f_2, each giving the probability of the respective genotype (with 0, 1, or 2 a alleles) developing the "abnormal" phenotype. The model usually assumes Hardy–Weinberg proportions, but this assumption can be relaxed by adding parameter(s). The SML model is quite general and includes classical Mendelian autosomal dominant and autosomal recessive models as subhypotheses. However, in the general model the terms *dominant* and *recessive* are not relevant.

General predictions for this model when $0 < f_i < 1$ for at least one f_i and $f_0 \leq f_1 \leq f_2$ include: (a) non-Mendelian patterns and frequencies in families and sets of families, (b) increased risk to subsequent siblings when families are ascertained through more than one affected sibling, (c) the risk to siblings and offspring of a proband will be greater than the risk to aunts/uncles or nephews/nieces and the risk will continue to decrease, approaching the population incidence asymptotically as the relationship to the proband becomes more remote, (d) if a sex or severity difference exists, it may be conceptualized as a different penetrance vector for each type and, when incorporated into the model, usually predicts that the less common type of proband will have a higher frequency of affected relatives than the more common type of proband. These are identical to the general expectations for the MFP model, as discussed by Mendell and Spence (1979).

A variety of methods have been proposed for estimating the parameters of the SML model. Using different analytic techniques it is possible to obtain parameter estimates from average frequency of affected relatives, from data on segregation in nuclear families, and from more extensive pedigrees. With familial prevalence data on a present/absent trait the parameters of the model cannot be uniquely specified (James, 1971; Kidd, 1975; Suarez, Reich, & Trost, 1976). Moreover, a goodness-of-fit test cannot be done and it can be shown that the SML and MFP models are actually only different parameterizations of the same mathematical relationship (Kidd & Gladstien, 1980).

Two-threshold models have also been developed for the SML model using severity (Reich et al., 1972) or sex differences (Kidd & Spence, 1976) to define the second threshold. These specific models were developed for application to data on pairwise frequency of disease and do allow goodness-of-fit tests. The MFP and SML two-threshold models are closely related (Kidd & Gladstein, 1980);

they evince differences only in the interrelationships of the various frequencies of affected relatives, and discrimination is possible with pairwise frequency data only if several different classes of relationship are studied. In applications to data on human disorders, discrimination has been less than perfect: For stuttering (Kidd, 1977) the models only differ appreciably in their predictions for the least frequently observed categories of relationships—relatives of female probands.

Analysis based on pairwise prevalences among relatives are not powerful, though it has been shown in simulations (Reich, Rice, Cloninger, Wette, & James, 1979) that the parameter estimates are not biased and are approximately correct if the data set is large. As these methods have the advantage of being reasonably simple to apply to a highly condensed tabulated data set, they are useful as an initial stage in an exploratory data analysis. However, any complete genetic analysis should eventually use much more powerful methods. Available methods can be conveniently divided into two general categories: complex segregation analysis and pedigree analysis.

Segregation is defined as the separation of alleles during meiosis. When the genetic model being tested is a simple Mendelian model, the expected ratios of genotypes is easily calculated and can quickly be compared to the observed ratios among the siblings of the affected probands. The expected ratios are conditioned on the most likely genotype of the parent given the specific genetic hypothesis. For simple traits, those which follow a Mendelian pattern, these analyses are sufficient. However, for complex traits (those traits which do not show a simple Mendelian pattern, e.g., speech and language disorders) additional parameters need to be added into the model and one relies more heavily on tests of genetic hypotheses under more general models rather than simple estimation of segregation ratios. This analysis allows estimation of the parameters of a specific model using nuclear family data and is known as segregation analysis.

Segregation analyses can give maximum likelihood estimates of the ascertainment probability and other parameters of the genetic model being used (Morton et al., 1971; Elandt-Johnson, 1970; Elston & Stewart, 1971). Statistical techniques can then be used to compare different hypotheses about the relationships of genotypes to phenotypes (e.g., if that relationship can best be explained by the MFP model or the SML model). The main drawback of most such analyses is that it must be assumed that all families included have the same genetic disorder and represent a random sample from a homogenous distribution of environments. For most common diseases, including speech and language disorders, both of those assumptions are questionable. Even the less restrictive models can accomodate only a limited amount of genetic heterogeneity.

Pedigree analysis using large multigenerational pedigrees is conceptually similar to segregation analysis of nuclear family data, but is generally considered more powerful because each pedigree contains more relationships. Specific hypotheses currently testable by pedigree analysis methods include single-locus inheritance, polygenic inheritance, and multilocus inheritance, among others (Elston & Yelverton, 1971; Lange & Elston, 1975; Lange et al., 1976; Elston & Namboodiri, 1977; Cannings, Thompson, & Skolnick, 1978). Parameters in the single-locus and multilocus models include the allele frequencies, the penetrances of all genotypes, and the transmission probabilities. Parameters in the polygenic model can include various components of variance—additive genetic, environmental, etc.—or more complex conditional transmission functions. A potential difficulty is that analyses of large pedigrees may be biased in favor of one specific hypothesis if only "interesting" pedigrees are analyzed. By establishing rules for the sequential sampling of pedigrees, it is possible to correct for such biases while avoiding unnecessary study of uninformative families (Cannings & Thompson, 1977).

The Mixed Model

Morton and MacLean (1974) have proposed another model which can be graphically represented in the same way as the single-major-locus model. However, the variation around genotype means is assumed to be in part polygenically inherited with a certain correlation among relatives. Thus, if both parents are heterozygotes at the upper end of the distribution for heterozygotes, their children will be distributed among the three main-locus genotypes as a result of Mendelian segregation but each will tend to be in the upper portion of his/her respective distribution because of the additive polygenic contribution to the liability. It is thus quite rightly referred to as the mixed model—it mixes together the multifactorial and the single-major-locus models. The model is not a model of heterogeneity as both systems contribute to the same liability.

The mixed model has several statistical advantages over either extreme model separately as both the MFP and SML modes are just special cases of the more general mixed model. Allowing the allele frequencies at the major locus to go to 0 and 1 causes the model to become identical to the multifactorial model. Allowing the polygenic–multifactorial correlations among relatives to go to 0 makes the model identical to the single-major-locus model. The nesting of each of the simple models into a general model allows a likelihood ratio test of either model to the full mixed model. However, as neither of the two extreme models is nested within the other, a direct comparison between them is not interpretable in terms of statistical significance.

STRATEGIES FOR THE STUDY OF SPEECH AND LANGUAGE DISORDERS

Several of the more common methodologies available for genetic analysis of complex disorders have been reviewed. A necessary first step in designing and conducting a genetic study for speech and language disorders is a general understanding of analytic methods available, of their data requirements, of the assumptions made, and of the specific answers obtainable with each method. It is necessary to know what questions can be answered and what types of data are necessary before a study can be designed and data collected. A general understanding of methods available will help in making decisions about experimental design. In the following paragraphs some of the considerations involved in making those decisions will be reviewed.

Because etiologic heterogeneity is such a likely phenomenon, the first consideration must be given to obtaining a sample that is as homogeneous as possible. One approach to minimizing heterogeneity is to exercise extreme care in selection of probands using diagnostic criteria that are as rigorous as possible. Indeed, it is possible to incorporate not only highly restrictive inclusion criteria but also very clear exclusion criteria so that probands represent an unusually clear diagnostic group. Although this group will not be representative of all affected individuals, it will be more likely to be homogeneous for a particular speech or language disorder. Generalization to the larger population will not be possible without qualification, but the information from the study of the families of such a group of probands should give insight into the study of other rigorously defined homogeneous proband samples.

After deciding upon a strategy for selection of a relatively homogeneous proband sample, the next step is to establish rigorous criteria for diagnosis of relatives. Although the criteria used for proband selection should also be used for relatives, other diagnostic categories need to be defined. It is unlikely that all affected relatives will meet the rigorous criteria used for proband selection—phenotypic expression is highly variable for speech and language disorders—and some allowance should be made for variation in expression. It is important that all criteria be established before data collection to avoid possible complications arising from changing diagnostic criteria after data have been examined.

In conjunction with determining the nature of the sample, it is necessary to formulate general hypotheses. Hypotheses of interest must be considered prior to data collection as different types of data may be appropriate for testing different hypotheses. Alternatively, if special circumstances dictate that only certain types of data will be available, noting which hypotheses might be studied with these data can assure that all relevant specific information is collected. The specific data collected should always include relevant diagnostic information but also might include biochemical data, genetic marker data for linkage analyses, and/or psychophysiological data.

In conclusion, the importance of hypothesis testing should be reemphasized: Understanding of a complex problem is advanced primarily by rejecting hypotheses (Popper, 1959). Because different types of data are suitable for testing different specific hypotheses, it is unlikely that any one study can, in itself, resolve the genetics of a speech or language disorder. However, that should not be a deterrent to further study. Each study will serve to reduce the range of reasonable hypotheses and increase their specificity.

REFERENCES

Cannings, C., & Thompson, E. A. Ascertainment in the sequential sampling of pedigrees. *Clinical Genetics*, 1977, *12*, 208–212.

Cannings, C., Thompson, E. A., & Skolnick, M. H. Probability functions on complex pedigrees. *Advances in Applied Probability*, 1978, *10*, 26–61.

Cavalli-Sforza, L. L., & Kidd, K. K. Genetic models for schizophrenia. *Neurosciences Research Program Bulletin*, 1972, *10*, 406–419.

Crittenden, L. B. An interpretation of familial aggregation based on multiple genetic and environmental factors. *Annals of the New York Academy of Sciences*, 1961, *91*, 769–780.

Elandt-Johnson, R. C. Segregation analysis for complex modes of inheritance. *American Journal of Human Genetics*, 1970, *22*, 129–140.

Elston, R. C., & Campbell, M. A. Schizophrenia: Evidence for the major gene hypotheses. *Behavior Genetics*, 1971, *1*, 3–10.

Elston, R. C., & Namboodiri, K. K. Family studies of schizophrenia. *Proceedings of the 41st Session of the International Statistics Institute*, 1977.

Elston, R. C., & Steward, J. A general model for the genetic analysis of pedigree data. *Human Heredity*, 1971, *21*, 523–542.

Elston, R. C., & Yelverton, K. C. General models for segregation analysis. *American Journal of Human Genetics*, 1975, *27*, 31–45.

Falconer, D. S. The inheritance of liability to certain diseases estimated from the incidence among relatives. *Annals of Human Genetics* (London), 1965, *29*, 51–76.

Gladstein, K., Lange, K., & Spence, M. A. A goodness of fit test for the polygenic threshold model. *American Journal of Medical Genetics*, 1978, *2*, 7–13.

James, J. W. Frequency in relatives for an all-or-none trait. *Annals of Human Genetics* (London) 1971, *35*, 47–49.

Kaplan, E. B., & Elston, R. C. *Program package for general pedigree analysis (GENPED)*. Unpublished Manuscript, 1976.

Kidd, K. K. On the possible magnitudes of selective forces maintaining schizophrenia in the population. In R. Fieve, D. Rosenthal, & H. Porill (Eds.), *Genetic research in psychiatry*. Baltimore: Johns Hopkins University Press, 1975.

Kidd, K. K. A genetic perspective on stuttering. *Journal of Fluency Disorders*, 1977, *2*, 259–269.

Kidd, K. K. Empiric recurrence risks and models of inheritance: Part II. In C. J. Epstein, C. R. Curry, S. Packman, S. Sherman, & B. D. Hall (Eds.), *Genetic counseling: Risks, communication and decision making*. New York: Alan R. Liss, 1979.

Kidd, K. K., & Gladstien, K. Alternative genetic models for the analysis of complex traits. In M. Melnick, D. Bixler, & E. D. Shields (Eds.), *Etiology of cleft lip and cleft palate*. New York: Alan R. Liss, 1980.

Kidd, K. K., & Spence, M. A. Genetic analysis of pyloric stenosis suggesting a specific maternal effect. *Journal of Medical Genetics*, 1976, *13*, 290–294.

Lange, K., & Elston, R. C. Extensions to pedigree analysis, I: Likelihood calculations for simple and complex pedigrees. *Human Heredity*, 1975, *25*, 95–105.

Lange, K., Westlake, J., & Spence, M. A. Extensions to pedigree analysis, II: Recurrence risk calculation under the polygenic threshold model. *Human Heredity*, 1976, *26*, 337–348.

Mendell, N. R., & Spence, M. A. Empiric recurrence risks and models of inheritance: Part I. In C. J. Epstein, C. R. Curry, S. Packman, S. Sherman, & B. D. Hall (Eds.), *Genetic counseling: Risks, communication and decision making*. New York: Alan R. Liss, 1979.

Morton, N. E., & MacLean, C. J. Analysis of family resemblance, III: Complex segregation of quantitative traits. *American Journal of Human Genetics*, 1974, *26*, 489–503.

Morton, N. E., Yee, S., & Lew, R. Complex segregation analysis. *American Journal of Human Genetics*, 1971, *23*, 602–611.

Popper, K. R. *The logic of scientific discovery*. London: Hutchinson, 1959.

Reich, T., James, J. W., & Morris, C. A. The use of multiple thresholds in determining the mode of transmission of semi-continuous traits. *Annals of Human Genetics* (London), 1972, *36,* 163–184.

Reich, T., Rice, J., Cloninger, C. R., Wette, R., & James, J. The use of multiple thresholds and segregation analysis in analyzing the phenotypic heterogeneity of multifactorial traits. *Annals of Human Genetics* (London), 1979, *42,* 371–389.

Suarez, B. K., Reich, T., & Trost, J. Limits of the general two-allele single locus model with incomplete penetrance. *Annals of Human Genetics* (London), 1976, *40,* 231–244.

IV

GENETIC COMPONENTS OF
COMMUNICATIVE IMPAIRMENTS

10

Linkage Analysis of Communication Disorders

WILLIAM J. KIMBERLING

Gene localization is concerned with the identification of the position in the genome of a segment of DNA and the characterization of that molecular variation which is represented by specific variation at the phenotypic level.

The importance of acquiring or creating a human gene map cannot be understated. If at the present time, our knowledge of the phenotype is less than extensive, our knowledge of the human gene map is even more limited. Of perhaps 100,000 genes, we have only a rough idea of the approximate positions of about 450 genes (less than 1%) and the base sequence of only a few such as the beta and alpha hemoglobin complexes and the insulin locus. In consequence, our ability to prevent and treat communication disorders is severely constrained.

GENERAL CONSIDERATIONS

In humans, the two principal methods of localizing genes are somatic cell genetics and classical linkage analysis.

Somatic cell genetics is ideally suited for localizing the genes that code for enzymes, cell surface antigens, and other factors that may be expressed in tissue culture. It is rapid and inexpensive. When human cells are fused with mouse cells, and cultured, human chromosomes are preferentially lost during the ensuing mitoses: If a particular human enzyme (or cell surface marker) is distinguishable from that expressed in the host cell, then clones of hybrid cells can be examined for the presence or absence of the human marker and this

151

GENETIC ASPECTS OF
SPEECH AND LANGUAGE DISORDERS

can then be correlated with the human chromosomes present in the clone and localization thereby achieved. As mentioned, the advantage of this method of gene localization is that it is rapid and inexpensive. The method also has several disadvantages:

1. The gene must be expressed in somatic cells (this excludes most dominant disorders).
2. The expression of the gene must be detectably different in the human versus the host.
3. The linear relationship of genes along the chromosome can only be determined by using cell lines with deleted portions of a human chromosome, and such abnormal chromosomes are not very common.

Somatic cell hybridization is not suited for localizing most autosomal dominant disorders (e.g., Waardenburg syndrome, Huntington disease) or for the study of more complex disorders such as dyslexia. In summary, somatic cell genetics, although a rapid and inexpensive method of localization, has only limited use in the study of human disease or behavior.

Classical linkage studies use large kindreds. The segregation of so-called marker (landmark) genes are examined in relation to the segregation of a given disease. Nonrandom assortment of the disease with one of the markers is indicative of linkage. If the marker has been localized to a chromosome, then the locus for the disease can be inferentially placed upon the same chromosome. This method is ideally suited for the gene localization of autosomal dominant traits which do not express their phenotype in cell cluture and may be useful in the study of human behavior disorders.

CURRENT STATUS OF THE CLASSICAL APPROACH TO GENE MAPPING

Linkage deals with the analysis of the segregation of alleles at two or more loci relative to one another. The original recognition of linkage was based on the discovery that certain pairs of genes did not segregate randomly with respect to one another, contrary to Mendel's second law of random assortment. This can be illustrated as follows. Assume, for example, two gene loci, A and B, each of which has two alleles: A_1, A_2 and B_1, B_2 respectively. Consider a mating of the type: A_1B_1/A_2B_2, so that all second generation offspring are of the type A_1B_1/A_2B_2. If such an offspring is backcrossed to someone with a genotype exactly like that of either of the parents, the mating can be represented symbolically as $A_1B_1/A_2B_2 \times A_2B_2/A_2B_2$. Four genotypes of third generation offspring are possible: A_1B_1/A_2B_2, A_2B_2/A_2B_2, A_1B_2/A_2B_2, and A_2B_1/A_2B_2. If A and B are unlinked, all four genotypes are equally likely. If A and B are linked, then the proportion of A_1B_2/A_2B_2 and A_2B_1/A_2B_2 offspring will diminish in proportion to the strength of the linkage.

Note that A_1B_1 and A_2B_2 represent grandparental genetic material transmitted from Generation 1 to Generation 3 "intact," that is to say that alleles from both A and B loci are both derived from either grandfather or grandmother but not both. The A_1B_2 and A_2B_1 gametes are termed recombinants and represent a new combination of genetic material derived from both grandmother and grandfather.

As already stated, the expectation is that all four gametes occur in equal proportion. Hence we would also expect a 1:1 ratio of recombinants to non-recombinants, or the fraction of recombinants of 50%. This recombination fraction, or 0, is defined as the number of recombinants over the total number of offspring.

For reasons that need not be detailed here, the recombination fraction is never expected to be greater than 50%. It is, however, frequently observed to be less than 50%. When the recombination fraction is less than one-half, this is evidence of nonrandom assortment and is usually due to linkage. Linkage is, in fact, nonrandom assortment of alleles from two loci because the loci are in close proximity to one another on the same chromosome.

At the chromosomal level, the mechanism of linkage is explained by the phenomenon of crossing over. Given two homologous chromosomes with loci A and B located at some distance from one another with alleles A_1 and B_1 on one homologue and alleles A_2 and B_2 on the other, the only way that B_1 and B_2 could come to lie on the same homologue is through a physical exchange of genetic material in the region between A and B. Chiasmata, which can be seen microscopically in meiotic cells, are felt to be physical representations of the crossover event. Crossing over is a biochemical process and occurs within fairly defined limits. In humans, for example, an average of 54 chiasmata are formed per meiosis (Hutten, 1974).

The distance between any two gene loci can be measured in terms of the recombination fraction. This distance will be roughly proportioned to the physical distance between loci. However, because the likelihood of crossing over is not evenly distributed across the genome, the correspondence between distance as measured by recombination fraction and the physical or actual distances is only approximate. Nonetheless, gene order should always correspond.

The following points about linkage should be kept in mind:

1. A recombination fraction of less than 50% is indicative of linkage.
2. Linkage between two loci implies that they lie on the same chromosome.
3. The recombination fraction is a rough measure of the phsycial distance between two chromosomes.
4. A recombination fraction of 50% indicates that the two loci are either on separate chromosomes or far apart on the same chromosome.

LIMITS OF GENE MAPPING

There are about 3.2×10^9 base pairs in the human genome. These base pairs constitute about 100,000 genes (Botstein, White, Skolnick, & David,

1980). Consequently, there should be about 3.2×10^4 (32 Kb) base pairs per gene, a number too large to agree with conventional estimates of gene size based on commonly accepted ideas of polypeptide size. This can be reconciled somewhat by postulating long inactive and/or repetitive sequences of DNA placed between the actual genes. This, plus only a two- to threefold underestimate of the number of genes, could easily explain this discrepancy. However, the number of genes and their average size in terms of number of base pairs is not really pertinent to the subject of localization. The important factor is the average number of base pairs to which a given gene can be localized with reasonable cost and effort. If, for example, a gene can be localized to a 10–20 Kb segment or less, then there will be a good likelihood of identifying and sequencing the actual gene responsible for a given disorder. The longer the segment, the less likely it is that such a one-to-one correspondence can be achieved.

A number of pragmatic factors have thus far limited the utility of family studies. These have to do with the number of landmark loci, their position in the genome, and the frequency of heterozygosity (i.e., frequency of informative matings) for each locus.

The distribution of the landmark loci is critical. The absolute minimum loci required per arm are two, one at the centromere (i.e., the constricted portion of the chromosome) and one at the telomere (i.e., the arm of the chromosome). For longer chromosome arms intermediate loci will be needed. Estimates indicate that about 80 such correctly positioned loci will be necessary to localize a test locus (2, 3). However, landmark loci are discovered randomly and their locations may not correspond at all with the ideal. A much larger number of markers may have to be screened before the ability to set up such an ideal set is achieved.

An important limitation is the frequency with which this set may be informative. This is dependent upon the number of alleles and their frequencies. Not every locus will be informative in every mating. A secondary set of markers will be required to ensure that information about every region is obtained from each meiosis.

With a sufficient set of primary and secondary markers, any gene should be localizable with reasonable accuracy and expense. We are possibly more than half way toward a sufficient set of markets. The centromeric heteromorphisms (i.e., polymorphic heritable differences at the centromere) tag the centromere and there are about 30 other markers available. The advent of restriction enzyme polymorphisms promises the rapid development of new markers (Goldgar & Kimberling, 1982).

The development of new marker loci is critical to future gene mapping in man. Because of the expense involved in acquiring samples, it is necessary to have as close to a 100% probability of finding linkage as possible. This can only be achieved by focusing first upon the development of a primary set of landmark loci.

FAMILY STUDIES

The classical approach to linkage requires the study of large multigeneration families. Given the current state of a limited number of genetic markers, most families are not large enough to provide a reasonable chance of finding linkage even if it does exist. The typical family is small and the number of possible observations is limited or critical individuals will be missing because of death or lack of cooperation. The lack of three-generation data complicates the analysis. Morton (1955) developed the lod score method of analysis, which was programmed by Ott (1974) to handle the difficult and varied types of analyses required in linkage investigations and in order to take advantage of all the information available from a family. Nonetheless, large families are required to ensure a reasonable probability of success. Usually, data from unrelated families must be pooled in order to achieve acceptable significance levels. This requires the assumption of homogeneity, that is to say that the disorder in each of the families is due to a mutation at the same locus. The assumption of homogeneity is not always warranted. Examples to the contrary include elliptocytosis (Morton, 1956), congenital cataract (Connealy et al., 1978) possibly spherocytosis (Kimberling, Taylor, Chapman, & Lubs), and dyslexia (Smith, Pennington, Kimberling, & Lubs,1980). When several small families constitute the sample, heterogeneity could conceal the fact of a loose linkage and by doing that also conceal the important fact of heterogeneity. The safest method of avoiding this problem is to study the very largest kindreds. This philosophy has restricted the families available for study. However, as the number of landmark loci increase, the need for such large families should decrease. Indeed, with a complete set of markers, only 5–10 observations are required to localize a gene to the equivalent of a band. Small families would then become useful enough to warrant their analysis as independent units.

A final point about family studies needs to be made. Taken individually, each genetic disease is rare. Some mutations such as private blood groups may occur exclusively in single families and represent the only opportunity to study the phenotypic effects of that gene. Others, such as Goldenhar syndrome, occur usually as sporadic cases and only rarely show a dominant pattern of inheritance. These families represent a resource which should be exploited. Full utilization requires the semipermanent storage of samples from these families so that localization can proceed as new markers become available.

UTILITY OF GENE MAPPING

Historically, geneticists have unraveled the underlying mechanisms of genetic disease by working "down," starting with the phenotype and gradually working backward along the pathogenetic chain to arrive at a hypothesized genotype. For example, phenylketonuria was described early as a possible subset of types of mental retardation with a characteristic and differentiable phenotype. The observation that this group had elevated levels of phenylalanine and its derivatives gave support to this initial classification and eventually led to observation that there were diminished levels of the enzyme that converted phenylalanine to tyrosine, phenylalanine hydroxylase. Even though, at this stage of the research, rational approaches of therapy could be formulated, it must be emphasized that all the observations are phenotypic. The gene defect must be inferred. The possibilities for the molecular defect are numerous: (a) the enzyme may be structurally altered and thereby by nonfunction; (b) the gene coding for the enzyme may be structurally absent due to a deletion; (c) a defect in control (extrinsic to the structural locus) may be the cause; and (d) the defect may be due to defective cofactor or some posttranslational control. There may be other possibilities. The point is that what appears to be a homogenous disorder at the phenotype level almost always will be more heterogeneous as one gets closer to the true basic defect, that is, the gene. This problem is compounded with communication disorders, which often appear heterogeneous at the phenotypic level. An understanding of heterogeneity is fundamental to the development of rational and effective strategies of treatment.

Furthermore, it should be realized that starting with only the phenotype and working backward along the etiologic steps is a cumbersome and lengthy proposition. It is possible with the new DNA technology to define the gene, in terms of its base sequence, and its phenotypic effect. If this is done, then the filling in of the intermediate causal steps should occur with greater rapidity.

REFERENCES

Botstein, D., White, R. L., Skolnick, M., & David, R. W. Construction of a genetic map in man using restriction fragment length polymorphisms. *American Journal of Human Genetics,* 1980, *32,* 314–331.

Connealy, P. M., Wilson, A. F., Merritt, A. D., Halveston, E. M., Palmer, C. G., & Wang, L. Y. Confirmation of genetic heterogeneity in autosomal dominant forms of congenital cataracts from linkage studies. *Cytogenetic Cell Genetics,* 1978, *22,* 295–297.

Goldgar, D. E., & Kimberling, W. J. Full information linkage analysis. In R. H. Jones (Ed.), *Medical application of statistics* (Vol. 1). 1982.

Hulten, M. Chiasma distribution at diakenesis in the normal human male. *Hereditas,* 1974, *76,* 55–67.

Kimberling, W. J., Taylor, R. A., Chapman, R. G., & Lubs, H. A. Linkage and gene localization of hereditary spherocytosis. *Blood,* 1978, *52,* 859–867.

Morton, N. E. Sequential tests for the detection of linkage. *American Journal of Human Genetics,* 1955, *7,* 277.

Morton, N. E. The detection and estimation of linkage between the genes for elliptocytosis and the Rhesus blood type. *American Journal of Human Genetics,* 1956, *8,* 80–96.

Ott, J. Estimation of the recombination fraction in human pedigrees: Efficient computation of the likelihood for human linkage studies. *American Journal of Human Genetics,* 1974, *26,* 588–597.

Smith, S. D., Pennington, B., Kimberling, W. J., & Lubs, H. A. Investigation of subgroups within specific reading disability utilizing neuropsychological and linkage analyses. *American Journal of Human Genetics,* 1980, *32,* 83A.

11

Dyslexia: Family Studies[1]

JOAN M. FINUCCI
BARTON CHILDS

INTRODUCTION

Previous Family Studies of Dyslexia

Familial reports of dyslexia or specific reading disability (SRD) include a wide variety of approaches. The simplest of these are reports of single families in which multiple cases occur. Such reports usually appear in the literature when a condition is first being described because familial occurrence is suggestive of a genetic explanation of at least some forms of the condition. Thus it was with dyslexia; several reports of aggregations of cases within one or two families (Fisher, 1905; Thomas, 1905; Hinshelwood, 1907, 1911; Stephenson, 1907) were made shortly after the first clinical description of the condition by Morgan (1896). An obvious bias is apparent in such single-family reports because they usually provide no account of how many isolated cases occur; but they do provide a stimulus for more systematic study of families.

Studies by Eustis (1947), Symmes and Rapoport (1972), and Rutter and Yule (1975) are illustrative of another approach. In each of these studies, one of the purposes was determination of familial incidence in families ascertained through a diagnosed dyslexic child. In each study the investigators, who had no prior knowledge of other affected members at the outset of the study, found a high incidence of reading disability in the families. This determination was made through interview data, however, rather than through objective measure-

[1]This work was supported by grants from the National Institutes of Health (HD 00486) and the Gow School.

157

ment techniques. The degree to which biases of the individual respondents (either underreporting or overreporting) affected the resulting familial incidence figures is not known. In none of these studies was there an attempt to examine patterns of transmission in families.

Another class of family studies compares the reading-related skills and other characteristics of relatives of disabled readers with those of relatives of normal readers. Typical of such studies are Owen, Adams, Forrest, Stolz, and Fisher (1971) and Foch, DeFries, McClearn, and Singer (1977). These studies showed poorer performance in the area of reading and spelling for the relatives of the disabled readers and, because of control of environmental factors, provided evidence for an important role of the genes in explaining familial incidence. But although objective measures of reading and spelling were obtained, no attempts were made to classify relatives as affected or unaffected. Thus, in these studies also, patterns of transmission within families could not be examined.

Hallgren's (1950) report is noteworthy because he studied a large number of families of disabled readers and because he not only attempted to determine the degree of familial aggregation, but he also statistically tested specific Mendelian hypotheses as explanations of patterns of transmission within families. His conclusion and that of a study by Zahalkova, Vrzal, and Kloboukova (1972), which was similar to Hallgren's but on a smaller scale, was that the transmission of dyslexia can best be explained by an autosomal dominant gene. Unfortunately, diagnoses given to most of the relatives relied heavily on reports by the subjects or their relatives, and although some test data were obtained, they were not always employed objectively. Furthermore, although Hallgren discussed the possible heterogeneity of reading disability, he treated his sample of families as a homogeneous group in testing genetic hypotheses.

All of these studies are significant because, although inconclusive with respect to the exact role of the genes in the origin of dyslexia, they are suggestive of some genetic involvement. That familial studies of dyslexia, so many years after its description, are wanting, reflects the general lack of agreement concerning procedures for objectively defining dyslexia in both children and adults, the dependence of genetic study of a behavior on procedures for defining that behavior, and the need for bringing several disciplines together to study the genetics of dyslexia.

Rationale for This Study

Our research group is studying families ascertained through a child with dyslexia with the purpose of determining if one or more forms of the condition can be accounted for by a specific genetic mechanism. Although our study falls within the domain of behavior genetics, the approach we take differs from that of many family and genetic studies of a behavior in that we are not interested in determining the heritability of dyslexia. Heritability, which is a measure of the importance of the genes relative to the environment in explaining the variance of a continuously distributed trait, is a group measure descriptive of the bulk of the cases in a distribution within a relatively homogeneous population. But it has little value in explaining the origin of cases at the extremes of a distribution where some cases may represent the outliers in a normal distribution, say, 1–2 standard deviations from the mean, and other cases, lying further from the mean, may arise from a specific event, either genetic or environmental, which has a major influence in determination of the trait; that is, these latter cases cannot be accounted for by the same factors that account for normal variation.

Rather, our research is based on the medical model, and our approach is allied to the methods used by Penrose (1965) and Roberts (1952) who studied families of children with mental retardation. We assume that dyslexia, like mental retardation, is heterogeneous both in its nature and in its cause. Furthermore, we assume that just as the majority of cases of mental retardation are multifactorial in origin with other cases arising from a variety of chromosomal or single gene effects, dyslexia may follow a similar pattern. Consequently, as a prelude to testing specific genetic hypotheses, one of our purposes is to identify attributes that may be used to characterize homogeneous subgroups of dyslexia in which those hypotheses may be tested. Beyond identifying these attributes, however, we are able to take advantage of the genetic method to test the validity of the attribute as a subgroup characteristic by examining within-family resemblance. The two aspects of our study that will be the focus of this chapter are definition and subgrouping.

DEFINITION

It is essential to our approach that the condition, dyslexia, be objectively defined and that its severity be quantified. We use a different measure for children and adults, but for both age groups (a) the measure may be treated either continuously or discretely, (b) the measure stems from the definition of dyslexia as "unexpected" reading disability, that is, achievement in reading and spelling that is discrepant from expected achievement, and (c) the measure is well validated by self-reports of reading and school history.

Quantitative Index for Children

For the children in our studies between grades 3 and 12, we derive an *achievement quotient* (Finucci, Isaacs, Whitehouse, & Childs, 1982), which is the ratio of achievement age as obtained from scores on the Gray Oral Reading Test and the spelling subtest of the Wide Range Achievement Tests (WRAT) to expected achievement age. The latter is the average of a child's chronological age, mental age, (determined from the WISC-R), and the average age of students at his grade placement. We use scores from oral reading and spelling tests rather than scores from silent reading comprehension tests because the former measure skills that are taught and are normally acquired early in a child's schooling. Deficits in those skills in an otherwise normally progressing child have been the classic symptoms for the diagnosis of dyslexia. Although comprehension deficits may accompany problems in word analysis and synthesis which would be noted on oral reading and spelling tests, it is our belief that difficulties in comprehension alone may stem from a more global cognitive problem rather than being confined to the area of reading.

We administer these tests and calculate quotients for all of the children in grades 3–12 in families ascertained through a disabled reader (the index case) and, in addition, we have done the same for 241 children in a comparison group in grades 3–12. These latter children attended parochial or public schools in middle- to upper-class neighborhoods similar to those in which our families of disabled readers reside. Approximately equal numbers of Caucasian boys and girls who spoke English as their native language were randomly sampled (with parental consent) for study without prior knowledge on our part of their reading and spelling ability.

Theoretically, children who achieve as expected should obtain quotients equal to 1.00; if better than expected, greater than 1.00; and if poorer than expected, less than 1.00. Benton (1975) suggested .80 as a point below which quotients are indicative of dyslexia. Myklebust (1968) included a milder affected region up through .90. Approximately 10% of the comparison group had quotients at or below .80 and an additional 17% had quotients between .81 and .90, which we refer to as a borderline region.

The distribution of quotients for the index cases is very different. All of the index cases in our study now attend or have attended special school programs for disabled readers, have a full-scale IQ of at least 95, and are free of severe psychiatric or sensory disorders. All of the cases we have tested who meet these criteria have had quotients at or below .90. For instance, among the 46 index

TABLE 11.1
Distribution of Achievement Quotients (AVQ) for 46 Index Cases
and 241 Comparison Children

	Index cases			Comparison children		
AVQ	N	%		AVQ	N	%
≤.60	5	(11)				
.61–.70	20	(43)				
.71–.80	13	(28)		≤.80	24	(10)
.81–.90	8	(17)		.81–.90	40	(17)
				≥.91	177	(73)
Total	46	(100)		Total	241	(100)

cases described in Finucci *et al.* (1982), the mean quotient is .71. Table 11.1 shows the contrast between the distribution of quotients for those index cases and the 241 comparison children.

We have validated the quotient as a measure of reading disability for children by relating it to responses to four multiple-choice questions concerning reading and school history. These items were given to all subjects after subjects had been administered the achievement and intelligence tests. We ask whether the subject had difficulty in learning to read, whether he had tutoring in reading, whether he repeated any grades, and what reading group he was in while in elementary school. Table 11.2 shows the relationship between the number of unfavorable responses to the four items and the values of the quotient for the 241 comparison children. Though the relationship is not a perfect one, 86% of those classified as normal readers gave no unfavorable responses, and only 17% of those classified as disabled readers gave no unfavorable responses. The distribution of unfavorable responses for the borderline subjects was intermediate to that for normal readers and that for disabled readers.

Further demonstration of the validity of the quotient is given by the responses of the 46 index cases. In this group, in which there was no one with a quotient above .90, the number of unfavorable responses to the history items, as well as to items relating to self-report of spelling ability and attitude toward reading, differed significantly from the comparison sample and increased as the value of the quotient decreased.

Quantitative Index for Adults

For an adult subject, the measure we use to describe reading and spelling ability is the average of the differences between predicted and obtained scores

TABLE 11.2

Number of Unfavorable Responses to Four History Items by Level of Quotient for Comparison Subjects[a],[b]

Number of unfavorable responses	Quotient					
	$\leq$ .80		.81–.90		$\geq$ .91	
	N	%	N	%	N	%
0	4	16.7	17	42.5	152	85.9
1	8	33.3	10	25.0	16	9.0
2	5	20.8	8	20.0	4	2.3
3	3	12.5	3	7.5	5	2.8
4	4	16.7	2	5.0	0	0.0
Totals	24	100.0	40	100.0	177	100.0

[a]From Finucci, Isaacs, Whitehouse, and Childs, 1982a, reprinted by permission of Spastics International Medical Publications.

[b]$\chi^2_{8df} = 84.47$, $p \leq .001$.

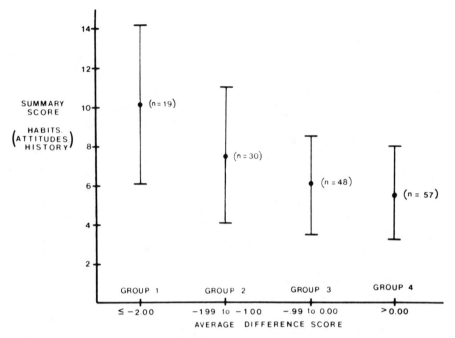

FIGURE 11.1. Means ±1 standard deviation of summary scores for 13 questions relating to reading habits and attitudes and reading and school history (four groups of adults divided according to average scores in reading and spelling).

on the Gray Oral Reading Test and WRAT spelling subtest. These difference scores are expressed in units of standard errors of prediction. The predicted scores for a subject are determined from multiple regression equations derived in a sample of adults between the ages of 18 and 65 who are similar to those in the families of index cases with respect to IQ, educational attainment, and socioeconomic status, but are not known to be related to a dyslexic child (Finucci, Whitehouse, Isaacs, & Childs, 1983, in press). The equations use sex, education, verbal IQ, and performance IQ as predictors.

Within the regression sample the average difference scores have the expected normal distribution about a mean of 0 with a standard deviation of 1. Among 154 adults in the families, however, there is a decided skewness toward negative scores. While only about $2\frac{1}{2}$% of the subjects would be expected to obtain scores 2 or more standard errors of prediction poorer than predicted, more than 12% of the 154 adults have scores at or below −2.00.

This adult measure is also shown to be valid by its relationship to self-reports of subjects. Figure 11.1 shows a plot of means and standard deviations of summary scores to 13 questionnaire items concerned with reading habits and attitudes as well as reading and school history. The higher the summary score, the poorer are a subjects's habits, attitudes, or history. When the 154 adults in the families are divided into four groups according to the value of their reading scores (Group 1 = poorest, Group 4 = best), those in Group 1 have significantly higher summary scores than do those in Group 2, who in turn have significantly higher scores than do those in Groups 3 and 4. Thus we consider adult scores at or below −2.00 as indicative of severe reading disability and scores greater than −2.00 and less than or equal to −1.00 as indicative of borderline reading disability.

CHARACTERISTICS FOR DESCRIBING SUBGROUPS

Severity

In his Galton lecture on the genetics of mental deficiency, Roberts (1952) discussed his hypothesis of multiple forms of mental deficiency. He suggested that one kind represented a single-factor, clear-cut difference from the normal, the sort of variation that interested Mendel; whereas another kind represented an extreme of continuous variation, the sort of variation that interested Galton. He added: "If there are indeed two kinds a recognition of that fact is quite the most important step in understanding how mental deficiency comes about. If we mix them up together we shall never get very far with our analysis [p. 71]." Roberts attempted to unscramble the mix using severity of mental retardation in index cases and their sibs as a subgrouping characteristic. He found that those families with the most severely retarded index cases whose sibs had a distribution of IQ more or less similar to that in the general population differed in a number of ways from the families of milder cases who had sibs with mild retardation also and who he suggested represented the tail end of the normal distribution of IQ. More of the latter group were drawn from the lower social classes which was probably just one of the factors contributing to the mild retardation.

We have also used severity as a measure in an attempt to sort out subgroups of dyslexia. For instance, we divided a group of 60 index cases into four subgroups according to the value of their achievement quotients. These subgroups are shown in Table 11.3. The two groups at the extremes—6 index cases with quotients at or below .60, and 11 index cases with quotients in the borderline region from .81 to .90—are clearly different from each other and from the two intermediate groups. Thus, as compared to the borderline subjects, the subjects with the lowest quotients (a) were on the average older (14.0 versus 10.0); (b) had a higher mean full-scale IQ (114 versus 104); (c) were more likely to have performance IQ higher than verbal IQ (50% of the cases versus 18% of the cases); and (d) had a higher proportion of dysphonetic spelling errors (54% versus 29%), a point that will be elaborated upon in the next section. The two groups with intermediate reading scores had values of these characteristics intermediate to those of the other two groups.

TABLE 11.3
Characteristics of 60 Index Cases Grouped by Severity

Variable	Group 1 ($N = 11$)	Group 2 ($N = 19$)	Group 3 ($N = 24$)	Group 4 ($N = 6$)
Quotient (range)	.81–.90	.71–.80	.61–.70	≤.60
Age ($\bar{X}$)	10.0	10.5	12.0	14.0
Full scale IQ ($\bar{X}$)	104	108	108	114
Subjects with performance IQ > verbal IQ (%)	18	21	29	50
PDP ($\bar{X}$)[a]	.29	.42	.44	.54

[a]PDP represents proportion of spelling errors that are dysphonetic.

Furthermore, the severe index cases have no severely affected parents, whereas the borderline subjects have both severe and borderline disabled parents. Also, the severe index cases have both disabled sibs and very normal reading sibs, whereas the borderline index cases have only borderline sibs. The parental and sib status of the most severe cases is suggestive of a recessive mode of inheritance but the borderline group may represent the end of a normal distribution in terms of developmental delay. They may simply "grow out of it" as they mature or it is possible that they are most responsive to remediation. We intend to examine this issue through follow-up testing.

Table 11.4 illustrates the relationship between severity of reading disability in parents and in their children. Data presented in the table represent the classification of school-age sibs listed according to parental scores from 60 families in which both parents were tested and in which the index case had school-age sibs. Although the most severe index cases had no severely disabled parents, the number of sibs affected at all varies as a function of the status of the parents. Also, in the three families in which both parents are disabled, two of four sibs are also disabled and the other two are borderline. These data illustrate

TABLE 11.4
Number of Affected Sibs According to Classification of Parents

Parental type	Number of families	Sibs			
		Normal	Borderline	Disabled	Total
At least one disabled (≤ -2.00)	13	7 (32%)	7 (32%)	8 (36%)	22
At least one borderline (-1.99 to -1.00)	22	23 (55%)	11 (26%)	8 (19%)	42
Both normal (> -1.00)	25	25 (64%)	10 (26%)	4 (10%)	39
Total	60	55	28	20	103

TABLE 11.5
Medians and Distributions of Proportion Dysphonetic Errors (PDP) of Offspring of
Reading-Disabled Parents Crosstabulated by Parental Value of PDP

PDP of affected parent	Median PDP of offspring	PDP of offspring				
		≤.24	.25–.49	.50–.74	≥.75	Total
≥.75	.76	0	2	1	4	7
.50–.74	.48	5	7	9	3	24
.25–.49	.33	1	4	1	1	7
≤.24	.25	4	3	2	0	9

the likelihood that most cases result from either a multifactorial or a dominant mode of transmission.

Together, the results of examining the status of parents and sibs according to the severity of the index cases and of examining the status of sibs according to the status of parents show the probable heterogeneity of cause of dyslexia.

Spelling Error Type

Another characteristic that we have used in an attempt to identify subgroups is the type of spelling error made by subjects when they misspell a word. Defining phonetic errors as those which may be pronounced to sound like the stimulus word and dysphonetic errors as those which when pronounced do not sound like the stimulus word, we have classified all of the errors made by our subjects in spelling the words in the WRAT spelling test as either phonetic or dysphonetic. Our scheme is a substantial modification of one proposed by Boder (1971). Using the scheme, we produce for each subject a measure, proportion of dysphonetic errors (PDP), which is an index of how dysphonetic his spelling is. Several authors have suggested that dysphonetic spellers have a deficit in processing or integrating auditory stimuli and represent a subtype of dyslexia (Boder, 1971; Camp & Dolcourt, 1977; Ingram, Mason, & Blackburn, 1970; Omenn & Weber, 1978).

In four groups of children, totaling 483 subjects and representing two groups of disabled readers and two groups of subjects selected without regard to reading ability, we have shown that PDP varies inversely with the value of the average achievement quotient in reading and spelling (Finucci, Isaacs, Whitehouse, & Childs, 1983). However, disabled readers do differ among themselves with respect to spelling error type, that is, some of the most severe mispell phonetically, lending strong support to the use of that characteristic for identifying subgroups.

Furthermore, there is intrafamilial likeness with regard to spelling error type. Table 11.5 gives the distributions and medians of PDP of reading-disabled offspring of reading-disabled parents according to the value of PDP of the affected parent. As indicated by the underscored numbers, the most frequent category for each row is that of the parental type. In addition, the median value for the offspring increases as the parental value increases. These data show that poor reading parents who misspell dysphonetically are more likely to have poor reading offspring who misspell dysphonetically than are phonetically misspelling parents; and poor reading parents who misspell phonetically are more likely to have children who misspell phonetically than are dysphonetically misspelling parents. Although this relationship can never be perfect, given the effort at schools to teach children to spell phonetically, this degree of within-family homogeneity attests further to the value of spelling error type for subgrouping.

DIRECTIONS FOR FUTURE RESEARCH

The attributes discussed—severity of dyslexia and type of spelling error—are only two of several characteristics that might be used to define subgroups of dyslexia. An important next step in genetic research will be to identify other characteristics that correlate with these two, as such identification would aid in further defining the subgroups. Possible candidates are reading comprehension patterns, Wechsler IQ factor scores, and measures of linguistic processes that have been shown to differentiate between normal and dyslexic adolescents (Whitehouse, 1982; Whitehouse & Moscicki, 1983). Only after these subgroups have been validated by showing within-family resemblance on the defining characteristics should tests of hypotheses of genetic transmission be undertaken.

In summary, this medical model shows some promise for differentiating cases and families. Its main drawback lies in the very large number of families required to reach definitive conclusions. There is a need for additional tests of attributes of language, and for tests of neurophysiological and biochemical distinctions, to enhance the discriminatory power of the model. As nearly every human phenotype studied has been shown to exhibit abundant heterogeneity, it is unlikely that this one will not.

REFERENCES

Benton, A. L. Developmental dyslexia: Neurological aspects. In W. J. Friedlander (Ed.), *Advances in neurology* (Vol. 7). New York: Raven Press, 1975.

Boder, E. Developmental dyslexia: Prevailing diagnostic concepts and a new diagnostic approach. In H. Myklebust (Ed.), *Progress in learning disabilities* (Vol. 2). New York: Grune & Stratton, 1971.

Camp, B., & Dolcourt, J. L. Reading and spelling in good and poor readers. *Journal of Learning Disabilities*, 1977, *10*, 46–53.

Childs, B., & Finucci, J. M. 1979. The genetics of learning disabilities. In R. Porter & M. O'Connor (Eds.), *Human genetics: Possibilities and realities.* New York: Excerpta Medica, 1979.

Eustis, R. Specific reading disability. New England Journal of Medicine, 1947, *237*, 243–249.

Finucci, J. M., Isaacs, S., Whitehouse, C., & Childs, B. Empirical validation of reading and spelling quotients. *Developmental Medicine and Child Neurology*, 1982, *24*, 733–744.

Finucci, J. M., Isaacs, S., Whitehouse, C., & Childs, B. Classification of spelling errors and their relationship to reading ability, sex, grade placement, and intelligence. *Brain and Language*, 1983, (In press).

Finucci, J. M., Whitehouse, C., Isaacs, S., & Childs, B. Derivation and validation of a quantitative definition of specific reading disability (SRD) for adults. *Developmental Medicine and Child Neurology*, 1983, (In press).

Fisher, J. Case of congenital word-blindness (inability to learn to read). *Ophthalmic Review*, 1905, *24*, 315–318.

Foch, T., DeFries, J., McClearn, G., & Singer, S. Familial patterns of impairment in reading disability. *Journal of Educational Psychology*, 1977, *69*, 316–329.

Hallgren, B. Specific dyslexia: A clinical and genetic study. *Acta Psychiatrica et Neurologica*, 1950 (Supplement 65).

Hinshelwood, J. Four cases of congenital word blindness occurring in the same family. *British Medical Journal*, 1907, *2*, 1229–1232.

Hinshelwood, J. Two cases of hereditary word-blindness. *British Medical Journal*, 1911, *1*, 608–609.

Ingram, T. T. S., Mason, A. W., & Blackburn, I. A retrospective study of 82 children with reading disability. *Developmental Medicine and Child Neurology*, 1970, *12*, 271–281.

Morgan, W. A case of congenital word blindness. *British Medical Journal*, 1896, *2*, 1378.

Myklebust, H. Learning disabilities: Definition and overview. In H. Myklebust (Ed.), *Progress in learning disabilities* (Vol. 1). New York: Grune & Stratton, 1968.

Omenn, G. S., & Weber, B. A. Dyslexia: Search for phenotypic and genetic heterogeneity. *American Journal of Medical Genetics*, 1978, *1*, 333–342.

Owen, F., Adams, P., Forrest, T., Stolz, L., & Fisher, S. Learning disorders in children: Sibling studies. *Monographs of the Society for Research in Child Development*, 1971, *36*, No. 4.

Penrose, L. *The biology of mental defect.* New York: Grune & Stratton, 1965.

Roberts, J. A. F. The genetics of mental deficiency. *Eugenics Review*, 1952, *44*, 71–83.

Rutter, M., & Yule, W. The concept of specific reading retardation. *Journal of Child Psychiatry*, 1975, *16*, 181–197.

Stephenson, S. Six cases of congenital word-blindness affecting three generations of one family. *Ophthalmoscope*, 1907, *5*, 482–484.

Symmes, J., & Rapoport, J. Unexpected reading failure. *American Journal of Orthopsychiatry*, 1972, *42*, 82–91.

Thomas, C. Congenital word-blindness and its treatment. *Ophthalmoscope*, 1905, *3*, 380–385.

Whitehouse, C. Token test performance by dyslexic adolescents. *Brain and Language*, 1983, *18*, 224–235.

Whitehouse, C., & Moscicki, E. *Nonsense word repetition and spelling by normal and dyslexic readers.* Manuscript submitted for publication, 1983.

Zahalkova, M., Vrzal, V., & Kloboukova, E. Genetical investigation in dyslexia. *Journal of Medical Genetics*, 1972, *9*, 48–52.

12

A Genetic Analysis of
Specific Reading Disability[1]

S. D. SMITH
B. F. PENNINGTON
WILLIAM J. KIMBERLING
H. A. LUBS

INTRODUCTION

The diagnosis of specific reading disability is generally made after exclusion of such obvious causes of reading problems as intellectual deficit, neurological abnormality, sensory handicap, lack of opportunity, or poor motivation. The resulting population is both clinically and etiologically heterogeneous and includes familial and sporadic cases. Because of this heterogeneity and the lack of precise diagnostic tests, convincing evidence for one or more modes of inheritance has not been forthcoming even though it has been reported that dyslexia is inherited in a dominant fashion in some families (Hallgren, 1950; Drew, 1956; Brewer, 1963; Zahalkova et al., 1972). Linkage analysis, as described in what follows, provides a unique means of defining a subgroup with a known genetic etiology by identifying and localizing a specific gene.

Background to Linkage Analysis

Two genes are said to be linked if they are inherited together more frequently than expected. By definition, both must be located close together on the same chromosome. In contrast, genes far apart on the same chromosome or on separate chromosomes will be transmitted in random combinations to the offspring. The degree to which the co-transmission of linked genes on the same chromosome deviates from randomness is expressed as the frequency of re-

---

[1]This work was supported by the National Institute of Health Grant HD13899.

169

combination, which is directly proportional to the distance between the genes. For example, 50% recombination represents random assortment, whereas 10% recombination would indicate that the genes are inherited together 90% of the time and thus are quite close together.

The probability of linkage, as determined by family studies, is computed for several recombination levels (θ); each probability is expressed as a lod score (log of odds of likelihood of linkage). Since they are a logarithmic expression of data, lod scores may be summed over families, for each value of θ, and the maximum lod score is taken to indicate the best estimate of θ. A maximum lod score greater than 3 has generally been considered sufficient to establish linkage, whereas a lod score less than -2 refutes linkage. The prior odds of a known gene being on a given chromosome are estimated to be 1 in 20; thus, the posterior probability of linkage with a lod score of 3 (odds of 1 in 1000) would be 1 in 50, which is an acceptable level of significance. In the present study, however, it could be argued that the assumption that we are dealing with a known gene is not met. We are, in fact, utilizing linkage to establish whether such a gene exists, so there would be no prior odds of linkage. A lod score of 3 then becomes more significant. Another important advantage of linkage analysis to the present study is the unlikelihood that misdiagnosis would produce a false positive result, since it should increase randomness and thus decrease the lod score (Morton, 1955).

Linkage analysis is thus able to overcome the problem of heterogeneity which has been one of the primary impediments in the study of reading disability, since individuals showing the same linkage necessarily have the same genetic etiology for their dyslexia. The clinical or behavioral findings in all families showing the same linkage can then be used to define the specific trait or disorder. Thus, for such a study, only the most basic initial definition of specific reading disability needs to be applied, since if linkage is found, further study of the phenotype will indicate which characteristics are actually a part of the individual disorder. Linkage analysis is also uniquely capable of detecting genetic heterogeneity. The example of elliptocytosis is a case in point. Two clinically identical forms have been separated through linkage studies, one linked to the Rh locus, the other not (Morton, 1956).

This study was designed to take advantage of these capabilities. Linkage analysis utilized known genetic markers for detection of a major gene, and two methods of classification of dyslexic subtypes were used for the phenotypic analysis. One system, developed by Mattis *et al.* (1975), classified dyslexics by neuropsychological characteristics, whereas the system of Boder (1973) is based on spelling errors.

METHODS

Ascertainment and Selection of Families

Families were selected in which specific reading disability appeared to be inherited in an autosomal dominant fashion so that linkage, if present, could be detected. Solicitation of families was through special schools and parents' groups. Those families which met certain initial criteria were interviewed. These included a proband with apparent specific reading disability and full scale IQ greater than 90 (initially determined from school records) and a parent and grandparent with a history of reading disability similar to that of the proband. Thus, only families with a positive family history over three generations were included in the study. Both parents and at least one sibling of the proband also had to be readily available for study. All families were Caucasian and native English-speaking.

An extensive family history was taken. The developmental and educational histories of the proband and sibs were reviewed, and appropriate medical and school records were requested. In families in which the history was compatible with specific reading disability and was transmitted in an autosomal dominant pattern, each member was asked to take a series of achievement tests.

Test Batteries and Diagnosis

An initial battery of diagnostic tests was administered. These were derived from two prior studies. Tests used by Finucci et al. (1976) included the Gray Oral Reading Test, the spelling subtest of the Wide Range Achievement Tests (WRAT), the transformed passages and nonsense passages. Tests recommended by the University of Colorado Family Reading Study included the Peabody Individual Achievement Test (PIAT: mathematics, reading recognition, reading comprehension, spelling, general information) and the Colorado Perceptual Speed Test (DeFries et al., 1978).

The usual definition of reading disability in children, a reading level at least 2 years below expected grade level, was used as the guideline for diagnosis. The Gray Oral Reading Test was used as the measure of reading ability, and the average of the PIAT mathematics and general information tests determined the expected level. In addition, a history of difficulty in school with reading and spelling was required. As the reading tests were sometimes inappropriate for adults, and because of the possibility of compensation, the primary criteria for the diagnosis of specific dyslexia in adults were pronounced difficulty in reading and spelling along with a positive family history.

If the results of these tests confirmed the diagnosis, all family members were given the tests shown in Table 12.1 and were included in the linkage analysis. This battery was not used in diagnosis, but was designed to replicate the work of Mattis et al. (1975) and Boder (1973). The test results were used to classify individuals into the Mattis et al. subtypes according to the criteria given in their paper. The Denver Reading and Spelling Test was designed by Camp and McCabe (unpublished) specifically to classify dyslexics according to Boder's formulations for dysphonetic and dyseidetic types. Classifications were examined for consistency within and between families.

Blood, urine, and saliva samples were obtained from all family members for linkage analysis. Phenotyping was done for 21 blood groups and enzyme

TABLE 12.1
Tests Used in Classification Battery

WISC-R or WAIS
Mattis Scheme
Language Disorder
  Boston Naming Test (E. Kaplan, H. Goodglass, S. Weintraub)
  Spreen-Benton Token Test
  Spreen-Benton Sentence Repetition Test
  Goldman-Fristoe-Woodcock Test of Auditory Discrimination
Articulation and graphomotor dyscoordination
  Goldman-Fristoe-Woodcock Sound Blending Test
  Graphomotor Test (Mattis *et al.*)
  Grooved Pegboard (Lafayette Instruments)
Verbal and NonVerbal Oral Expression (H. Goodglass, E. Kaplan)
Visuospatial perceptual disorder
  Raven's Progressive Matrices (adapted by University of Colorado)
  Benton Test of Visual Retention
  Primary Mental Abilities Test of Spatial Rotation
Boder Scheme
  Denver Reading and Spelling Test (L. McCabe, B. Camp)

markers (Table 12.2) as well as for chromosomal Q and C band heteromorphisms (Figure 12.1). Linkage analysis was done with the computer program LIPED by J. Ott (1974). After our preliminary results suggested linkage with chromosome 15, only chromosomal heteromorphisms were typed.

RESULTS

Twelve kindreds comprising 105 individuals were found to fit our criteria after being given the diagnostic battery of tests, and four additional families

TABLE 12.2
Genotyping Markers

ABO	Adenosine deaminase (ADA)
Rh	Esterase D (EsD)
MNS	Salivary amylase (Amy 1)
Kell	Pancreatic amylase (Amy 2)
Kidd (Jk)	Transferrin (Tnf)
Duffy (Fy)	Haptoglobin (Hp)
P	Group specific component (Gc)
Gm immunoglobulin	Phenothiocarbamide (PTC) taster (Ta)
Acid phosphatase 1 (A_{21})	Tongue rolling (Tr)
Phosphoglucomutase (PGM_2)	Secretor 1 (Sec 1)
6-Phosphogluconate dehydrogenase (6PGD)	

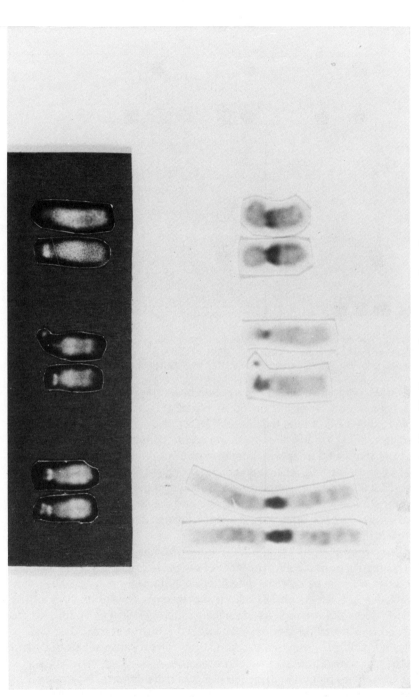

FIGURE 12.1. Samples of Q- and C-band heteromorphisms. The D group chromosomes shown illustrated the variations in fluorescent intensity seen with Q-banding, and C-band size variations are demonstrated by representative chromosomes 1, 15, and 16.

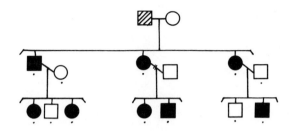

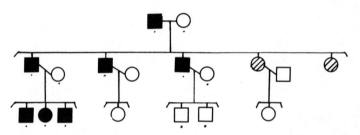

FIGURE 12.2. Two sample pedigrees. Dots beneath symbols indicate individuals included in the study. Blackened symbols indicate individuals with specific reading disability, while cross-hatching indicates those who were affected by history but who could not be tested.

have been ascertained and are being tested. Genotyping and chromosomal analysis have been completed on 80 individuals. Two sample pedigrees are shown in Figure 12.2. A total lod score of 3.241 at $\theta = .13$ has been obtained for specific reading disability and chromosome 15 heteromorphisms (Table 12.3). (Note that one family was uninformative for chromosome 15 so a lod score is not available.) All other markers produced lod scores less than 1.0. To eliminate bias in reading chromosome 15 markers in the remaining individuals, cytogenetic studies are now analyzed blindly, and the code is broken only when an entire family has been analyzed. As a result, linkage data are available only for nine families.

As can be seen from Table 12.3, Family 432 has a particularly high lod score. This results from the large number of people (15) studied in this kindred, and does not indicate a biological difference. In contrast, Family 491 has a very negative lod score which could indicate nonlinkage. As the analysis of the overall lod scores did not indicate significant heterogeneity ($\chi^2 > .05$), we are not justified in eliminating this negative lod score from the total. The distinct possibility remains, however, that this family may have a different type of dyslexia, with the locus being on another chromosome.

The presenting picture in these families was quite uniform. No evidence of any problems other than in reading and writing were detected in the history, the school records, the medical records when they could be obtained, or in our

TABLE 12.3

Lod Scores for Specific Reading Disability and Chromosome 15 Heteromorphisms[a]

0 Family	.00	.05	.10	.20	.30	.40
371	.602	.535	.465	.318	.170	.049
372	∞	−.350	−.126	.019	.043	.027
375	.903	.836	.766	.612	.438	.237
484	.602	.535	.465	.318	.170	.049
576	.301	.258	.215	.134	.064	.017
491	∞	−1.885	−1.076	−.377	−.081	.026
432	2.755	2.501	2.237	1.673	1.060	.414
005	.301	.258	.215	.134	.064	.017
Total	∞	2.688	3.161	2.831	1.928	.836
			3.241 at θ = .13			

[a]Scores are given for each family at different values of theta (θ), the recombination fraction. By interpolation, a maximum score of 3.241 is obtained at θ = .13.

observations. As in previous studies, males were generally more severely affected than females by history, and the abnormalities were often more difficult to detect in adults, particularly female adults. Figures 12.3 and 12.4 give examples of the handwriting and spelling from individuals from two families. There appeared to be a concentration of occupations in the building trade. Affecteds, however, included both a physician and lawyer, and one female English teacher.

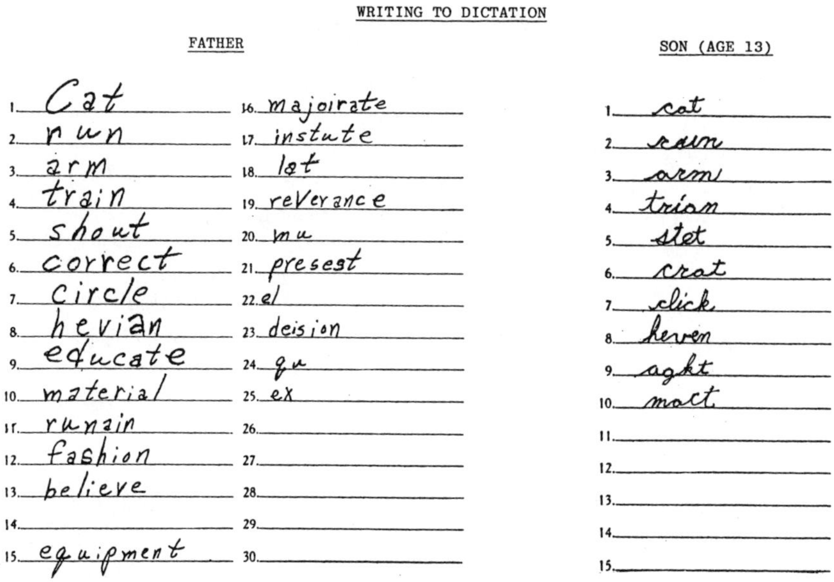

WRITING TO DICTATION

FATHER

SON (AGE 13)

FIGURE 12.3. Spelling samples from a man and his 13-year-old son.

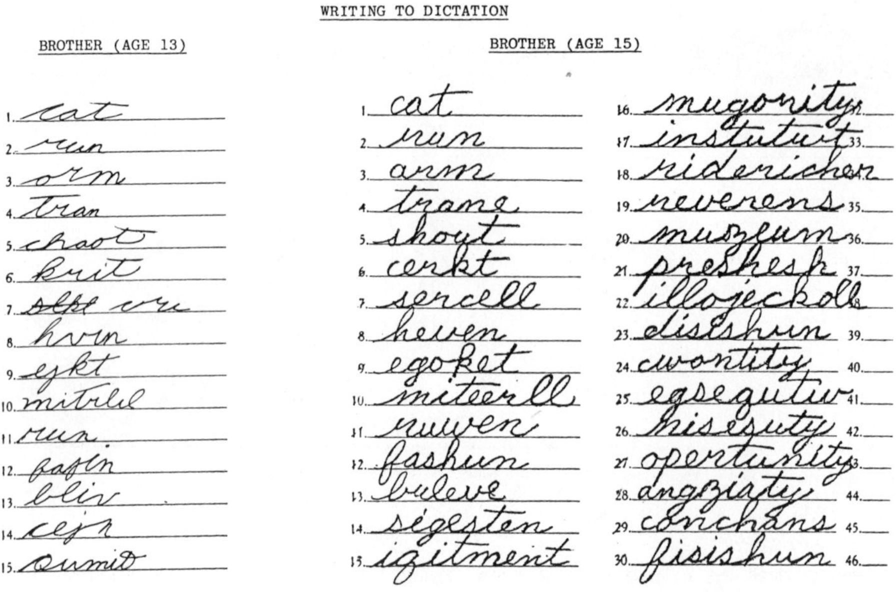

WRITING TO DICTATION

FIGURE 12.4. Spelling samples from two brothers.

When the results of the neuropsychological classification were used to classify individuals into the subtypes defined by Mattis *et al.* (1975), only 6 out of the 43 affected individuals tested were found to fit into any of the subtypes. All six of 43 were classified as having a language disorder. Thus, the vast majority of dyslexics did not show characteristics of any of the subtypes. Analyses of variance of the individual test scores using age as a covariate indicate that the only tests showing a significant difference between affecteds and unaffecteds were the Weschler Digit Span, Boston Naming test, and the noise subtest of the auditory descrimination test.

The results of the Boder spelling analysis were similar, in that over half of the affecteds were classified as having normal spelling patterns. The remainder were classified as dyseidetic, indicating that most of their errors showed ability to use phonetic analysis. Moreover, there was no familial consistency in classification as "normal" or "dyseidetic." However, further analysis of the spelling phenotype has shown the dyslexics produce significantly fewer phonetic equivalent misspellings; hence, their classification as dyseidetic is misleading (Pennington *et al.*, 1982).

DISCUSSION

A lod score of 3.241 strongly suggests linkage between a major gene influencing dyslexia and chromosome 15p heteromorphisms. Confirmation by a second study is required before a linkage is considered proven. Alternatively, a significant lod score between dyslexia and the hexosaminidase A locus on the distal long arm of chromosome 15 would provide confirmation. This, however, would require the study of a large number of Jewish families with dyslexia, and the data may be difficult to obtain. Approximately 1 person in 30 of Ashkenazy Jewish decent is heterozygous at this locus. Many such heterozygotes, however, have been ascertained through Tay–Sachs screening programs and could be screened secondarily for a history of dyslexia.

Within the present study group, the Boder and Mattis typing clearly are not useful. Very likely the composition of both study groups was different from ours, as our study population was not derived from clinical referrals.

The results of the Mattis test battery indicate that the deficits in the dyslexics in these families are primarily confined to reading and spelling. Visuoperceptual and motor abilities are grossly normal, but more sophisticated or physiological tests might demonstrate a significant defect. Further analysis of spelling errors suggests that there are developmental differences in acquisition of phonetic strategies (Pennington *et al.*, 1982). The consistent finding of only reading and spelling problems in affected family members further demonstrates that the deficit is quite specific in this type of dyslexia. Certainly, our data indicate that significant reading and spelling problems can exist in the absence of the gross neuropsychological deficits seen in other subtypes. These findings would be consistent with a gene affecting a circumscribed structure or function within the brain. This approach, therefore, offers the opportunity of studying the effects of a single mutant gene on an important function of the brain.

CONCLUSIONS

1. The linkage and family approach presented here have proven extremely fruitful and are applicable to many other behavior genetics problems characterized by heterogeneity and complications in diagnosis. Critical aspects of such studies include selection of families and test batteries as well as the application of linkage analysis itself.

2. With the currently available battery of markers, there is a 50–80% probability of identifying close linkage if one exists. Such studies cannot be considered "fishing expeditions," as many still consider linkage studies to be, but rather studies with a high probability of obtaining the desired information.

3. A gene playing a major role in this type of specific reading disability has tentatively been localized to chromosome 15, and the disorder appears to be inherited as an autosomal dominant trait. Preliminary identification of a distinct entity has also been accomplished, and an etiology has been assigned to one subgroup of dyslexic children. These children had only reading and writing disabilities and no other evidence of intellectual or motor problems.

4. The results also suggest the possibility of a phenotypically similar disorder not due to a gene on chromosome 15.

5. Further work is clearly indicated, including studies of the early development of reading abilities in affected families, long-term follow-up, ascertainment of more families to delineate additional entities, and the development of improved, simpler, and shorter tests, including a possible screening test. Neurophysiological studies and studies that might better delineate the functional nature of the abnormality are also needed. A unique opportunity to study the effects of one gene on information processing has evolved from these studies.

REFERENCES

Boder, E. Developmental dyslexia: A diagnostic approach based on 3 atypical reading–spelling patterns. *Developmental Medicine and Child Neurology,* 1973, *15,* 663–687.

Brewer, W. F. Specific Language Disability: Review of the literature and family study. AB Honors Thesis, Harvard College, 1963.

DeFries, J. C., Singer, S. M., Foch, T. T., Lewitter, F. I. Familial Nature of Reading Disability. *British Journal of Psychiatry* 1978, *132,* 361–367.

Drew, A. L. A neurological appraisal of familial congenital word-blindness. *Brain,* 1956, *79,* 440–460.

Finucci, J. M., Guthrie, J. T., Child, A. L., Abbey, H., Childs, B. The genetics of specific reading disability. *Annals of Human Genetics* (Lond) 1976, *40,* 1–23.

Hallgren, B. Specific dyslexia "cogenital word-blindness": A clinical and genetic study. *Acta Psychiatrica et Neurologica Supplement* 65.

Mattis, S., French, J. H., Rapin, I. Dyslexia in children and young adults: 3 independent neuropsychological syndromes. *Developmental Medicine and Child Neurology* 1975, *17,* 150–163.

Morton, N. E. Sequential tests for the detection of linkage. *American Journal of Human Genetics,* 1955, *7,* 277–318.

Morton, N. E. The detection and estimation of linkage between the genes for elliptocytosis and the RH blood type. *American Journal of Human Genetics,* 1956, *8,* 80–96.

Ott, J. Estimation of the recombination fraction in human pedigrees: efficient computation of the likelihood for human linkage studies. *American Journal of Human Genetics,* 1974, *26,* 588–597.

Pennington, B. F., McCabe, L., Smith, S. D., Kimberling, W. J., Lubs, H. A. An analysis of spelling errors in familial dyslexics. Paper presented to International Neuropsychological Society, Pittsburgh, Pennsylvania, February, 1982.

Zahalkova, M., Vrzal, V., Klobovkova, E. Genetical investigations in dyslexia. *Journal of Medical Genetics,* 1972, *9,* 48–62.

13

Sex Chromosome Abnormalities and the Development of Verbal and Nonverbal Abilities[1]

C. NETLEY

In this chapter evidence is presented which indicates that abnormal numbers of X chromosomes are associated with selective impairments in verbal or nonverbal abilities. Although most of the research to be described has been conducted with genetically abnormal individuals, its implications are not necessarily confined to these subjects and, indirectly at least, bear on questions of theory debated in other contexts. Before these issues are discussed, a review of the findings supporting an association between the X chromosome and the specific components of intelligence is presented.

SOME BASIC OBSERVATIONS

The commonest but least convincing form of evidence for an association between the sex chromosomes and abilities is derived from studies of normal 46 XY males and 46 XX females, many of which have indicated a male superiority on spatial tasks and a female advantage on verbal ones (Bock, 1973; Maccoby & Jacklin, 1974). Such results are consistent with an association between the specific components of ability and sex chromosomes but, of course, do not provide conclusive evidence for such a relationship. Somewhat more persuasive are studies that have examined patterns of correlations for specific abilities between parents and children. In some cases, these have indicated that the correlations between the spatial skills of different-sex combina-

---

[1]The work presented in this chapter has been supported by the Ontario Mental Health Foundation.

GENETIC ASPECTS OF
SPEECH AND LANGUAGE DISORDERS

tions (e.g., father and daughter) are higher than those between same-sex combinations (e.g., father and son) and, as a result, have prompted hypotheses concerning an X-linked mode of inheritance for this ability (Stafford, 1961; Bock & Kolakowski, 1973). The empirical evidence in support of such theories has been inconsistent, however (DeFries, Ashton, Johnson, Kuse, McClearn, Mi, Rashad, Vandenberg, & Wilson, 1976; Loehlin, Sharon, & Jacoby, 1978), and the proposal remains essentially unproven (see Vandenberg and Kuse, 1979, for a review of this area).

There has been little research directly concerned with possible genetic mechanisms underlying the frequently observed female superiority on verbal tasks. Lehrke (1974) studied individuals with generalized retardation and severe degrees of language disability and proposed that the verbal impairments in these cases could be accounted for by an X-linked mode of inheritance. This hypothesis does not, however, explain the verbal superiority of normal females.

Research with aneuploid subjects who have abnormalities in sex chromosome complement provides the most direct evidence for a relationship between cognitive functioning and the sex chromosomes. Turner syndrome (TS) females, who have a 45 X complement, have been shown repeatedly to have deficits in spatial or nonverbal functioning despite normal levels of verbal skills (Garron, 1977; Money, Alexander, & Walker, 1965; Netley, 1977; Rovet & Netley, 1980; Shaffer, 1962). Several studies have also indicated that males and females with a supernumerary X (i. e., with a 47 XXY or 47 XXX complement) have specific impairments in verbal skills. Although some of these studies have examined clinically identified patients (e.g., Garvey & Mutton, 1973), perhaps the most compelling evidence for verbal deficits in these subjects has been obtained from groups identified in neonatal screening programs where possible subject selection biases are minimized. Several such studies have been carried out and in those which have prospectively examined intellectual development there has been a remarkable consistency, with most indicating that 47 XXY males and 47 XXX females have circumscribed limitations in verbal abilities (Robinson, Lubs, Nielsen, & Sorensen, 1979). The nonverbal abilities of these subjects have usually been average or near average. Interestingly, there is little evidence to suggest that the Y chromosome has a comparable effect on intellectual functioning (Robinson et al., 1979).

Our studies of extra X males and females have been carried out with subjects identified by Bell and Corey (1974) in a neonatal screening study conducted in Toronto between 1967 and 1972. In this survey only one 45 X female was found, and as a result our investigations of this type of subject have been done primarily with cases identified because of clinically evident disorders of growth or endocrine functioning. A summary of the results of intellectual testing of the three kinds of X aneuploid subjects we have studied is presented in Table 13.1.

These data provide support for two conclusions. The first is that anomalous numbers of X chromosomes appear to impair the development of either

TABLE 13.1
WISC-R Test Results for 45 X, 47 XXY, and 47 XXX Children

		45 X ($N = 35$)	47 XXY ($N = 34$)	47 XXX ($N = 11$)
Verbal IQ	Mean	97.5	84.5	83.7
	SD	15.8	14.9	11.2
Performance IQ	Mean	84.4	101.1	96.9
	SD	14.6	12.3	12.9

verbal or nonverbal abilities. The second, more intriguing implication is that the relationship between chromosomal state and intellectual functioning is asymmetrical in the sense that the absence of a normally occurring X interferes with one area of functioning (nonverbal) whereas the presence of a supernumerary X depresses a different ability (verbal). These findings have led us to examine a number of different issues, which can be formulated in terms of the following questions:

1. What is the nature of the cognitive impairments in subjects with X aneuploid conditions?
2. What form of theory is most appropriate to explain the intellectual deficits of X chromosome aneuploid subjects?
3. What mechanisms are responsible for mediating the relationship between biologically defined chromosomal abnormalities and the intellectual disorders of individuals with X aneuploid conditions?

Each of these issues is examined in the following sections.

THE NATURE OF THE COGNITIVE DISORDERS IN FORTY-FIVE X AND EXTRA X SUBJECTS

Most of the evidence presented thus far has been derived from standardized psychometric tests. Such instruments are reasonably satisfactory for establishing the existence of intellectual disorders, but do have limitations in specifying the mechanisms that underlie these disorders. They do not, for example, provide much insight into whether the cognitive disorders seen in subjects with chromosomal anomalies are due to abnormalities in the cognitive strategies they use to solve verbal and nonverbal tasks. This issue is not much clarified by studies that have employed procedures which have some psychodiagnostic value in other clinical contexts. Commonly, investigations of this sort use what can be called the "lesion analogue" form of inquiry. Money (1973), for example, reported that TS individuals showed some (but not all) of the impairments found in patients with right parietal lobe lesions and on this basis argued that they had a similar neural defect. Silbert, Wolff, and Lilienthal (1977) observed that TS cases were deficient on tests thought to be dependent on right-hemisphere function and proposed a generalized disorder at this locus as the etiological agent. Waber (1979) interpreted her finding that TS subjects have particular difficulties with tests of fluent production as indicating a frontal lobe disorder.

Studies such as these are flawed for two reasons. The first concerns the logic of attributing neural deficits to TS subjects on the basis of their similarity to patients with demonstrated neural lesions. Evidence from other techniques sensitive to neurological integrity (CT scans, EEGs, etc.) would seem to be a minimum requirement before such inferences could be drawn, and even then other explanations, not involving putative lesions, are quite possible. The second weakness of such studies is that they usually do not provide any more insight into the processes or mechanisms underlying the cognitive disorders than do the psychometric instruments that are used to describe them.

The assumption that we have made is that procedures drawn from cognitive psychology can be particularly useful in arriving at an understanding of the intellectual impairments seen in the chromosomally abnormal. For example, in our investigation of 45 X TS females we were concerned with determining whether performance differences between these subjects and normal females were qualitative and as well as quantitative in kind. The results of an experiment using the "mental rotation" paradigm developed by Shepard and his colleagues (Shepard & Metzler, 1971) indicated that TS subjects and controls could be distinguished only in such quantitative terms as accuracy and speed in solving spatial problems. No qualitative differences in performance could be identified suggesting that, although less efficient than normal females, TS subjects use essentially normal strategies in dealing with spatial tasks (Rovet & Netley 1980, 1982).

In the case of extra X subjects, our research into the nature of their intellectual deficits has focused on the question of whether these individuals have primary disorders of short-term memory (STM) of the kind seen in learning disabled children. This possibility was suggested by the marked similarities in the intellectual and educational characteristics of these two kinds of subjects. Both perform poorly academically and usually share specific limitations in verbal ability (Netley, 1981). Since there is evidence that STM deficits may underlie the verbal disorders of learning disabled children (Cohen & Netley, 1978) we conjectured that the verbal disorders of extra X children may also be based on limitations in STM functions.

Our investigations of this issue are described elsewhere (Stewart, Bailey, Netley, Rovet, Park, Cripps & Curtis, 1982) and are presented here only in summary form. In these studies two sets of controls for each aneuploid group were employed, one matched for WISC-R Verbal IQ (CI) and the other for Performance IQ (C2). This use of two control groups provided us with the opportunity to assess the contribution of the lower-than-average verbal abilities

TABLE 13.2
WISC-R Test Results for 47 XXY Male and 47 XXX Female Samples and Verbal-IQ-Matched (C1) and Performance-IQ-Matched (C2) Controls

	N	Mean age	Mean Verbal IQ	Mean Performance IQ
Males				
47 XXY	34	10.2	84.5	101.1
C1	32	10.4	85.6	99.7
C2	34	10.4	111.2	102.5
Females				
47 XXX	10	9.9	82.4	96.5
C1	10	9.8	86.8	97.3
C2	10	9.7	97.7	99.7

of the aneuploid subjects to whatever STM deficiencies were found. The ages and intellectual characteristics of all groups are presented in Table 13.2.

The dependent variables were derived from either fairly simple descriptive tests of span length or more experimental procedures drawn from the cognitive psychology literature. The results, which are summarized in Table 13.3, indicate that the extra X male and female subjects performed less well than the controls in the span tests and also in most of the experimental conditions. In our original article we drew several conclusions:

> These results provide support for the view that STM impairments are present in extra X subjects and cannot be explained simply on the basis of limitations in verbal intelligence. Secondly, while other factors may also be involved, it appears that deficiencies in maintaining the strength of the memory trace are responsible for at least part of their recall disorders. Finally, we believe that the results support the view that language processing deficits compound or exacerbate any primary pre-linguistic deficiencies in recall that these subjects have [Stewart, Bailey, Netley, Rovet, Park, Cripps, & Curtis, 1982, p. 142].

WHAT FORM OF THEORY BEST EXPLAINS THE COGNITIVE DEFICITS OF ANEUPLOID CHILDREN?

Several kinds of explanations, each suggested by research with chromosomally normal subjects, might be considered relevant to an understanding of the cognitive deficits of X chromosome aneuploids. For example, it might be thought that gender-specific socialization processes, which may be responsible for some of the intellectual differences between normal males and females (Nash, 1979), could explain the findings with chromosomally abnormal subjects. However, theorizing in these terms does not readily account for why

TABLE 13.3

Summary of Studies of Short-Term Memory in 47 XXY and 47 XXX Subjects and Controls[a]

Test	Procedure	Results
Span length	WISC-R digit span and WPPSI sentences subtests.	47 XXY and 47 XXX subjects performed at lower levels than both sets of controls ($p < .05$).
Recall of verbal and spatial information	Based on a paradigm devised by Salthouse (1975) requiring the poststimuli cued recall of either verbal or spatial information.	47 XXY and 47 XXX subjects obtained lower levels of performance in all conditions ($p < .01$) compared to both sets of controls.
Probed serial recall of visual information	Based on a procedure developed by Wagner (1978) which requires subjects to recall the position of specified items in a serial array.	47 XXY males obtained lower scores than either set of controls ($p < .05$). 47 XXX females scored lower than C1 controls ($p < .05$) but not the more intelligent C2s.
Probed serial recall of auditory information	A 9-digit list is presented by audiotape and followed by a letter (A, B, or C) which specifies which third of the series is to be reported. Based on research by Cohen and Sandberg (1977) and Cohen and Netley (1978).	47 XXY males recalled fewer items from the last third of the materials than either set of controls ($p < .05$). They also recalled fewer items from the first third than C2 controls ($p < .01$). 47 XXX females reported fewer digits from all thirds of the lists than their C1 controls ($p < .05$).
Unrehearsed STM ability	This task required subjects to report the last three digits of lists of unpredictable length. Presentation rates vary from 1.75 to 8 digits per sec (Cohen & Netley, 1978).	Both aneuploid groups reported fewer digits than either set of controls with all rates of pesentation ($p < .05$).

[a]For details, see Stewart, Bailey, Netley, Rovet, Park, Cripps, and Curtis, 1982.

phenotypic females with a 47 XXX complement have essentially identical deficits in verbal ability as phenotypic males with a 47 XXY constitution (Netley, 1980). Moreover, socialization does not provide an explanation for the clearly different cognitive impairments of phenotypic females with 45 X and 47 XXX constitutions. A further difficulty arises from the fact that the severity of the specific intellectual deficits seen in these subjects is generally greater than those observed in chromosomally normal males and females (Rovet & Netley, 1979).

Finally, mention can be made of a study of a pair of dizygotic twins, one of whom was a 45 X TS and the other a normal 46 XX female (Rovet & Netley, 1982). These girls were subject to quite similar environmental influences which, under a socialization theory, would be expected to produce similar patterns of ability. In fact, the 45 X TS girl exhibited the usual spatial deficit whereas her twin did not.

Alternative explanatory possibilities for the specific impairments of X chromosome aneuploids are suggested by theories concerning the influence of sex hormones on normal intellectual development. For example, it has been proposed that normal sex differences in ability are due to the actions of the prenatal sex hormones which produce the distinguishable phenotypes of males and females. These, it is held, have additional consequences in influencing brain development in ways that create functional differences between the sexes in neural organization and abilities (see Reinisch, Gandelman, & Speigel, 1979). However, two points lead one to question the relevancy of this to findings obtained from children with abnormal numbers of X chromosomes. The first is that 47 XXY boys and 47 XXX girls have essentially identical deficits in verbal function despite having experienced sufficient differences in prenatal sex hormones to result in their separate phenotypic development as males and females. In addition, girls with 45 X and 47 XXX chromosome constitutions both lack androgens (although they presumably differ in estrogen levels) yet show quite different kinds of intellectual deficits. Other theories concerning the influence of sex hormones at puberty on ability (Petersen, 1979) also appear inadequate in relation to much of the data obtained with X aneuploid children as it is clear that their cognitive deficits exist before puberty and in the absence of any hormonal abnormality (Robinson et al., 1979; Stewart, Bailey, Netley, & Haka-Ikse, 1978).

Research conducted by Waber (1976, 1977a, 1977b) provides a different perspective on the issue of the biological determinants of specific intellectual abilities. She investigated chromosomally normal males and females who were either delayed or advanced in the onset of puberty and found that maturation rate was significantly related to the relative development of verbal and nonverbal skills. Her findings indicated that, regardless of sex, slow developers were more able spatially than verbally, whereas early maturers, again regardless of sex, tended to be more competent verbally than spatially. These findings suggested the possibility of some parallels between Waber's study groups and aneuploid subjects. Her slow developers and extra X subjects both, of course, are relatively weak verbally, whereas, her fast developers and 45 X cases have specific deficits in spatial functioning. There are several reasons to believe that these groups share similarities in other areas as well. It is known, for example, that growth rates as indicated by bone age assessments are delayed in extra X subjects (Stewart, Netley, Bailey, Haka-Ikse, Platt, Holland, & Cripps, 1979). It has also been reported that the index of growth hormone activity provided by the sulphation factor is elevated in 45 X females (Almqvist, Lindsten, & Lindvall, 1963).

Perhaps most significant are findings indicating that rates of mitotic cell division are abnormal in X aneuploid subjects, being higher than expected in 45 X females and lower than expected in extra X males and females (Barlow, 1973; Mittwoch, 1973). Taken together, these findings suggest that the patterns of atypical growth and intellectual deficit seen in X chromosome aneuploid subjects correspond to those reported by Waber in her investigations of pubescent subjects.

We have conducted several studies of the apparent association between growth and intellectual functioning in X aneuploid subjects. In the first we examined the relationship between growth rates, as indicated by bone age determinations, and the ability patterns of 45 X, 47 XXY, and 47 XXX subjects. The results of comparisons between these groups were consistent with the conclusion the degree of bone age retardation in relation to stature is correlated with the extent to which verbal ability falls below nonverbal ability (Stewart et al., 1979). Our second study was more stringent and was done by assessing whether the severity of bone age retardation was associated with the degree of verbal impairment *within* groups of 47 XXY and 47 XXX subjects. The results were positive, as the findings indicated that the children who were most verbally impaired were those with the most severe degrees of bone age dysmaturity (Netley & Rovet, 1982a).

Finally, we carried out a study that suggests a relationship between prenatal growth rates and the intellectual characteristics of X chromosome aneuploids. In this investigation we made use of the index of prenatal growth rate that is provided by total dermal ridge counts (TDRC) of the fingers. Dermal ridges differentiate by mid-fetal-life and do not change after this point (Holt, 1968). A high TDRC is thought to indicate a faster than normal fetal growth rate, whereas a low count indicates a slow fetal growth rate (Barlow, 1973; Mittwoch, 1973). As would be expected, the TDRCs of 45 X females are higher than average and those of 47 XXY and 47 XXX subjects are lower than average (Penrose, 1967; Hzrecko & Sigmon, 1980). In our study of children with a supernumerary X, we found that those with the lowest TDRCs had the greatest deficits in verbal intelligence and were most impaired on a sentence–picture verification task of language comprehension (Netley & Rovet, 1982a).

These findings are similar to those obtained by Waber (1976, 1977a) in general terms but differ from hers in one major respect. Her data were obtained from pubescent subjects whereas our aneuploid subjects, who were approximately 9 years of age, were without any signs of pubertal onset by clinical or endocrinological examinations (Stewart et al., 1979). The implication, of course, is that theorizing cast in terms of mechanisms operative at puberty, which Waber was led to, need not apply to aneuploid subjects. In their case, whatever mechanism is responsible for an association between patterns of growth and intellectual abilities must be due to events that have their effects well before this time. Indeed, given the relationship observed between the index of prenatal growth and the degree of verbal disability in extra X cases the implication is that the process is one that is initiated not long after conception.

MECHANISMS RELATING GROWTH TO INTELLECTUAL DEVELOPMENT IN X CHROMOSOME ANEUPLOIDS: A HYPOTHESIS

The material reviewed thus far provides some support for the proposition that disturbances in growth underlie the intellectual deficits seen in children with abnormal numbers of X chromosomes. It does not, however, shed much light on how these effects occur. This issue is addressed in this section.

Several lines of evidence suggest that an analysis of the neural bases of cognition is a worthwhile point to begin in any attempt to explain the relationship between biological and psychological development in individuals with abnormalities in sex chromosome complement. Some of this is provided by studies of normal males and females using such experimental procedures as dichotic listening or half-field tachistoscopic projection in which verbal or nonverbal stimuli are presented separately to lateralized sensory channels. Normal subjects when tested in these ways frequently show asymmetries in performance such that stimuli presented to one body side are more accurately reported than the same kind of material presented to the other. A common result when verbal stimuli are used is that material presented to right-sided sensory channels is better processed than that which goes to the left. In the case of nonverbal material the converse is usually found (Bryden, 1979). The most frequently advanced explanation for these observations is that each is the result of the superior transmission capacities of contralateral projection systems as compared to ipsilateral ones combined with the left hemisphere's specialization for verbal processing and the right's for nonverbal or spatial processing (Witelson, 1977).

The evidence for the relevance of investigations using these procedures to subjects with anomalous numbers of X chromosomes is provided by reports that indicate that normal males and females perform differently on laterally presented tasks. McGlone and Davidson (1973), for example, found that females tend to show a greater right-field advantage for tachistoscopically presented dots than males. Kimura (1969) obtained a similar result, while Witelson (1976) reported that males show a left-hand advantage on a dichhaptic nonverbal task earlier than girls. These and other results using the dichotic listening procedure (although the evidence using this technique has been variable; (see Witelson, 1977) have frequently been interpreted to indicate that males are more hemispherically specialized than females (Bryden, 1979, Waber, 1977b).

Additional evidence in support of this conclusion is found in the literature on the differential effects of brain lesions on males and females. For example,

Lansdell (1968) reported that right temporal lobectomies had a more disruptive effect on the spatial abilities of males than females. Furthermore, he found that only in the case of the male patients was it possible to demonstrate a correlation between the degree of spatial impairment and the amount of lost neural tissue. McGlone and Kertesz (1973) reported that the spatial impairments of females were related to the severity of their verbal deficits suggesting that they employ left-hemisphere-based verbal strategies for spatial tasks, whereas males use right-hemisphere nonverbal processes. McGlone (1977) provided additional evidence on this question in her study of unilaterally brain-damaged males and females. She found that males had greater verbal deficits with left-sided lesions than females and concluded they were more hemispherically specialized. She suggested that the cerebral hemispheres of females were less specialized with both contributing to verbal and nonverbal functioning.

Although these results obtained with chromosomally normal males and females are consistent with the view that the sex chromosomes influence hemispheric organization they do not, of course, provide any conclusive form of evidence. Somewhat more persuasive in this regard are the results of studies in which the hemispheric organization of subjects with abnormal numbers of sex chromosomes are examined. Several investigations of 45 X females have indicated that these individuals perform atypically on a verbal dichotic listening test. Each has demonstrated that the 45 X subjects are less likely than normal females to show the expected right-ear advantage in reporting dichotically presented material (Netley, 1977; Netley & Rovet, 1982b; Waber, 1979). Moreover, in one (Netley & Rovet, 1982b), it was found that those 45 X females without ear asymmetries were those with the most severe impairments of nonverbal ability.

Although these results support the possibility that abnormalities in numbers of X chromosomes may affect hemispheric organization and intellectual functioning, they do not make clear how these effects occur. The hypothesis we would propose is designed to deal with the following considerations: Disturbances in growth of individuals with anomalous numbers of Xs begin early in life and probably depend on deviations in mitotic cell division rates; the cognitive deficits of these subjects are apparent during childhood and cannot plausibly be explained by abnormalities in socialization processes or by disorders in hormonal functioning either prenatally or during adolescence; finally, relationships exist between the degree of pre- and postnatal growth delay and the severity of verbal disability in extra X subjects. Although much is missing in this network of findings which could provide support for our hypothesis, it is offered in part for its heuristic possibilities some of which we have examined and report in what follows.

Our initial assumption is that the growth rates of X chromosome aneuploids differ from those of normal males and females. If the atypical somatic growth rates that characterize individuals with a supernumerary or absent X chromosome are assumed to affect neural development from conception, then it follows that the brains of these individuals would be different from normals in

TABLE 13.4
Phi Coefficients of 47 XXY Boys and IQ- and Age-Matched Controls

Task	47 XXY ($N = 32$)	Controls ($N = 97$)	p
Half-field dot enumeration[a]	Mean = .122	.023	$p < .01$
Dichotic CVs[b]	Mean = .060	.100	$p < .01$

[a] Scored as left > right.
[b] Scored as right > left.

some growth-related parameter even during fetal life. (This inference is supported by studies that indicate a positive relationship between rates of neural and epidermal growth; e.g., Shaumann & Alter, 1960). A second necessary assumption is based on the work of investigators who have studied the anatomical bases of intellectual functioning. Wada, Clarke, and Hamm (1975) and Witelson and Paillie (1973) have provided evidence for the existence of an area in the left cerebral hemisphere, identifiable in the perinatal period, which probably or possibly subserves later language development. If this left temporal area is relatively mature at birth, it would be expected that verbal development would proceed without complication. Conversely, if immature, language would be expected to be delayed. Levy (1969) has proposed that the development of hemispheric specialization for verbal and nonverbal abilities arises because of a competitive interaction between these functions for the available neural tissue. Her formulation suggests that this antagonistic, competitive process may be biased in one direction or the other depending on the relative states of verbal and nonverbal development. In the case of 45 X females—who are fast developers, as indicated by mitotic cell division rates and TDRCs (see earlier discussion)—the neural sites for language development would be relatively mature and verbal functions diffusely represented in both hemispheres. Their nonverbal deficits would arise, therefore, from a diminished right-hemisphere capacity for such functions. This explanation suggests 45 X Turners would have less hemispheric specialization than normals and so be less asymmetric on such tasks as dichotic listening. As already mentioned, several studies using this technique have reported just such a result (Netley, 1977, Netley & Rovet, 1982b; Waber, 1979).

The explanation for the verbal deficits of 47 XXY boys and 47 XXX girls begins with the inference that their slower-than-average growth rates would delay the maturation of left-hemisphere-based language acquisition sites. Verbal development would occur slowly and so minimally interfere with the right hemisphere's capacity to establish nonverbal abilities. For these subjects it would be predicted that hemispheric asymmetries would be exaggerated. We have examined this prediction in several studies of 47 XXY boys using lateralized stimulus presentation paradigms such as dichotic listening for CVs and tachistoscopic dot and letter recognition tasks. The controls in this study were

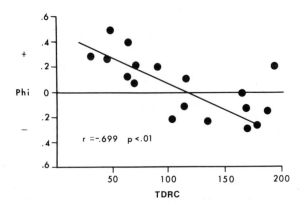

FIGURE 13.1. Asymmetries in dichhaptic test performance as a function of total dermal ridge counts (TDRC) in 18 47 XXY boys (positive phis reflect left-hand advantages).

IQ- and age-matched normals. The findings, which are presented in Table 13.4, are in part as predicted since they show a greater left-field advantage in the tachistoscopically presented dot enumeration task for the aneuploids than for the controls. In the case of dichotically presented CV material the results are not as expected since the aneuploids show a smaller mean asymmetry in performance than do the controls. These results suggest a modification of one aspect of our hypothesis. It is conceivable that the delayed growth of 47 XXY cases' left-hemisphere language sites permits the development of the right hemisphere's nonverbal and verbal abilities to a greater degree than normal, with the result that asymmetries are small for verbal stimuli and large for nonverbal stimuli. If so, the verbal deficits observed in these subjects could be the result of these functions being partially represented in their inherently linguistically less competent right hemispheres.

We have also conducted studies into an additional implication of our neurodevelopmental model. These studies were based on the inference that if the prenatally initiated growth delays of extra X males and females permitted the greater development of right-hemisphere sites concerned with spatial processes, then correlations should be found between individual differences in prenatal growth rates and indices of right-hemisphere spatial specialization. In particular, it would be expected that those subjects with the slowest growth would be those with the greatest degrees of left-sided advantage for bilaterally presented nonverbal tasks. The results of recognition studies employing tachistoscopically presented dots and dichhaptically presented shapes are shown in Figures 13.1 and 13.2 and are consistent with this prediction.

PROBLEMS AND UNANSWERED QUESTIONS

The material presented provides some support for the proposition that the specific intellectual deficits observed in individuals with anomalous numbers of

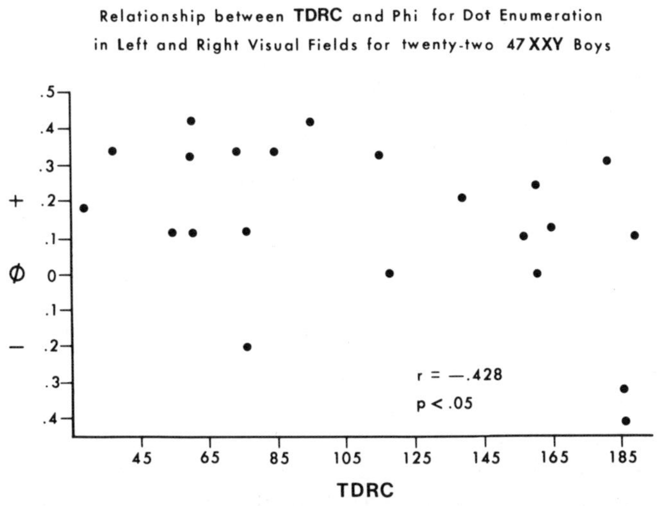

Relationship between **TDRC** and **Phi** for Dot Enumeration
in Left and Right Visual Fields for twenty-two **47 XXY** Boys

FIGURE 13.2. Asymmetries in performance on a half-field tachistoscopically presented dot enumeration task as a function of total dermal ridge counts in 22 47 XXY boys (positive phis reflect superior performance for left-field stimuli).

X chromosomes are due to disturbances in maturational processes, beginning early in life, which affect functional neural organization and the development of abilities. Needless to say, much more experimentation is necessary before this hypothesis can be regarded as even provisionally established. There is an obvious need, for example, to examine relationships between individual differences in rates of growth, intellectual functioning, and hemispheric organization in 45 X TS females. However, even if the general thrust of the ideas advanced here were to be accepted as correct, a number of questions remain unanswered. One of these concerns the functional significance of the Y chromosome. Penrose (1967), after surveying the literature on X and Y aneuploid subjects, observed that the relations between mean TDRC and the X and the Y chromosomes were similar, in that additional instances of either an X or a Y depressed TDRCs. However, the effect of an extra Y was only one-third that of an extra X. This suggests that individuals with a 47 XYY complement would have similar deficits to those with a 47 XXY constitution but to a less extreme degree. The evidence on this question is scanty at present, although the collated material reported by Robinson et al. (1979) provides some support for the conclusion that 47 XYY males are at risk for language disorders.

There is a further question concerning the course of language development in extra X subjects. It is unclear from the available evidence whether at maturity these individuals achieve normal levels of competence in verbal abilities. Given that the nonverbal deficits of 45 X TS females typically do not diminish as the individuals mature (Nielson, Nyberg, & Dahl, 1977), it is perhaps most reasonable to expect that the verbal disorders of extra X subjects will also persist. Only studies of mature subjects will provide a definitive answer to this question.

Aside from these matters, there is an additional issue which in its simplest terms concerns the relationship between the intellectual disorders observed in the chromosomally abnormal and those seen in patients with no demonstrable genetic anomaly. Are the disorders similar phenotypically and, perhaps more importantly, do they depend on the same mechanism of disordered growth? At this point, although the answer to the first aspect of this question is a tentative "yes," the answer to the second aspect remains completely uncertain. At present, only the work of Schlager, Newman, Dunn, Crichton, and Schulzer (1979) indicating that delays in bone age development are frequently found in the learning disabled suggests that similar processes may operate in euploid and aneuploid cases.

One problem in extrapolating from the chromosomally abnormal to the normal is exemplified by the following. It is well recognized that developmental disorders of language are much commoner among males than females (Rutter, Tizard, & Whitmore, 1970), yet, contrary to our hypothesis concerning the influence of prenatal growth, the mean TDRC of males is higher than that of females. Although this sex difference may be due to the higher incidence of arches in females than males, which would have the effect of spuriously lowering TDRCs in females (Holt, 1968), this explanation is clearly post hoc and the issue remains. At present, it can only be concluded that the concept of disturbed growth rates may provide a useful focus for future investigations into the origins of developmental disorders in verbal and nonverbal abilities.

ACKNOWLEDGMENTS

The writer is grateful for the invaluable contributions of his colleague, Dr. Joanne Rovet, and our research assistants, Valdine Dewan and Jeannine Pinsonneault, to the research program.

REFERENCES

Almqvist, S., Lindsten, J., & Lindvall, N. Linear growth, sulfation factor activity and chromosomal constitution in 22 subjects with Turner's syndrome. *Acta Endocrinologica,* 1963, *42,* 168–186.

Barlow, P. The influence of inactive chromosomes on human development. *Humangenetik,* 1973, *17,* 105–136.

Bell, A., & Corey, P. A sex chromatin and Y body survey of Toronto newborns. *Canadian Journal of Genetics and Cytology,* 1974, *16,* 239–250.

Bock, R. Word and image: Sources of the verbal and spatial factors in mental test scores. *Psychometrika,* 1973, *38,* 437–457.

Bock, R., & Kolakowski, D. Further evidence of sex-linked major gene influence on human spatial visualizing ability. *American Journal of Human Genetics,* 1973, *25,* 1–14.

Bryden, P. Evidence for sex-related differences in cerebral organization. In M. Wittig & A. Peterson (Eds.), *Sex-related differences in cognitive functions.* New York: Academic Press, 1979.

Cohen, R., & Netley, C. Cognitive deficits, learning disabilities and WISC verbal performance consistency. *Developmental Psychology,* 1978, *14,* 624–634.

Cohen, R., & Sandberg, T. Relation between intelligence and short-term memory. *Cognitive Psychology,* 1977, *9,* 534–554.

DeFries, J. C., Ashton, G. C., Johnson, R. C., Kuse, A. R., McClearn, G. E., Mi, M. P., Rashad, M. N., Vanderberg, S. G., & Wilson, J. R. Parent–offspring resemblance for specific cognitive abilities in two ethnic groups. *Nature,* 1976, *261,* 131–133.

Garron, D. Sex linked recessive inheritance of spatial and numerical abilities and Turner's syndrome. *Psychological Review,* 1977, *77,* 147–152.

Garvey, M., & Mutton, D. E. Sex chromosome aberrations and speech development. *Archives of Diseases in Childhood,* 1973, *48,* 937–941.

Holt, C. *The genetics of dermal ridges.* Springfield, Ill.: Thomas, 1968.

Hzrecko, T., & Sigmon, B. The dermatoglyphics of a Toronto sample of children with XXY, XXYY and XXX aneuploidies. *American Journal of Physical Anthropology,* 1980, *52,* 33–42.

Kimura, D. Spatial localization in left and right visual fields. *Canadian Journal of Psychology,* 1969, *23,* 445–448.

Lansdell, H. Effect of extent of temporal lobe ablations on two lateralized deficits. *Psychology and Behavior,* 1968, *3,* 271–273.

Lehrke, R. X-linked mental retardation and verbal disability. *Birth Defects: Original Article Series,* 1974, *10,* whole number.

Levy, J. Possible basis for the evolution of lateral specialization of the human brain. *Nature,* 1969, *224,* 614–615.

Loehlin, J., Sharon, S., & Jacoby, R. In pursuit of the "spatial gene": A family study. *Behaviour Genetics,* 1978, *8,* 27–42.

Maccoby, E., & Jacklin, C. *The psychology of sex differences.* Stanford: Stanford University Press, 1974.

McGlone, J. Sex differences in the cerebral organization of verbal functions in patients with unilateral brain lesions. *Brain,* 1977, *100,* 775–793.

McGlone, J., & Davidson, W. The relation between cerebral speech laterality and spatial ability with special reference to sex and hand preference. *Neuropsychologia,* 1973, *11,* 105–113.

McGlone, J., & Kertesz, A. Sex differences in cerebral processing of visuo-spatial tasks. *Cortex,* 1973, *9,* 313–320.

Mittwoch, U. *Genetics of sex differentiation.* New York: Academic Press, 1973.

Money, J. Turner's syndrome and parietal lobe functions. *Cortex,* 1973, *9,* 385–393.

Money, J., Alexander, D., & Walker, H. *A standardized road-map test of directional sense.* Baltimore: Johns Hopkins University Press, 1965.

Nash, S. Sex role as a mediator of intellectual functioning. In M. Wittig & A. Peterson (Eds.), *Sex-related differences in cognitive functioning.* New York: Academic Press, 1979.

Netley, C. Dichotic listening of callosal agenesis and Turner's syndrome patients. In S. Segalowitz & F. Gruber (Eds.), *Language development and neurological theory.* New York: Academic Press, 1977.

Netley, C. *Cognitive development, cerebral organization and the X chromosome.* Paper presented at the NATO, Advanced Study Institute on Neuropsychology and Cognition, Augusta, Georgia, September 1980.

Netley, C. *Prenatal and postnatal growth as predictive factors in educational disorders.* Paper presented at the Gatlinburg Conference on Developmental Disorders, Gatlinburg, Tennessee, March 1981.

Netley, C., & Rovet, J. Verbal deficits in children with 47,XXY and 47,XXX karyotypes: A descriptive and experimental study. *Brain and Language,* 1982, (a) *17,* 58–72.

Netley, C., & Rovet, J. Diminished hemispheric specialization of Turner syndrome subjects. *Cortex,* 1982, (b) *18,* 377–384.

Nielsen, J., Nyberg, H., & Dahl, G. Turner's syndrome. A psychiatric-psychological study of 45 women with Turner's syndrome, composed with their sisters and woman with normal karyotypes, growth retardation and primary amennorrhea. *Acta Jutlandica XLV, Medicine Series,* 1977, *21,* Arhus.

Penrose, L. Finger print patterns and the sex chromosomes. *Lancet,* 1967, *1,* 298–300.

Petersen, A. Hormones and cognitive functioning in normal development. In M. Wittig & A. Petersen (Eds.), *Sex-related differences in cognitive functioning.* New York: Academic Press, 1979.

Reinisch, J., Gandelman, R., & Spiegel, F. Prenatal influences on cognitive abilities: Data from experimental animals and human genetic and endocrine syndromes. In M. Wittig & A. Petersen (Eds.), *Sex-related differences in cognitive functioning.* New York: Academic Press, 1979.

Robinson, A., Lubs, H., Nielsen, J., & Sorensen, K. Summary of clinical findings: Profiles of children with 47,XXY, 47,XXX and 47,XYY karyotypes. *Birth Defects: Original Article Series,* 1979, *15,* 261–266.

Rovet, J., & Netley, C. Phenotypic vs genotypic sex and cognitive abilities. *Behaviour Genetics,* 1979, *9,* 317–322.

Rovet, J., & Netley, C. The mental rotation task performance of Turner syndrome subjects. *Behaviour Genetics,* 1980, *10,* 437–443.

Rovet, J., & Netley, C. Processing deficits in Turner's syndrome. *Developmental Psychology,* 1982, *18,* 77–94.

Rutter, M., Tizard, J., & Whitmore, K. *Education, health and behaviour.* London: Longmans, 1970.

Salthouse, T. A. Simultaneous processing of verbal and spatial information. *Memory and Cognition,* 1975, *3,* 221–225.

Schlager, G., Newman, D., Dunn, H., Crichton, J., & Schulzer, M. Bone age in children with minimal brain dysfunction. *Developmental Medicine and Child Neurology,* 1979, *21,* 41–51.

Shaffer, J. W. A specific cognitive deficit observed in gonadal aplasia (Turner's syndrome). *Journal of Clinical Psychology,* 1962, *18,* 403–406.

Shaumann, B., & Alter, M. *Dermatoglyphics in medical disorders.* New York: Springer-Verlag, 1960.

Shepard, R. N., & Metzler, J. Mental rotation of three-dimensional objects. *Science,* 1971, *171,* 701–703.

Silbert, A., Wolff, P. H., & Lilienthal, J. Spatial and temporal processing in patients with Turner's syndrome. *Behaviour Genetics,* 1977, *7,* 11–21.

Stafford, R. E. Sex differences in spatial visualization as evidence of sex-linked inheritance. *Perceptual and Motor Skills,* 1961, *13,* 428.

Stewart, D., Bailey, J., Netley, C., & Haka-Ikse, K. *Indications for X and Y chromsome surveys.* Paper presented at the meeting of the Canadian Pediatric Society M, Halifax, 1978.

Stewart, D., Bailey, J., Netley, C., Rovet, J., Park, E., Cripps, M., & Curtis, J. A. Growth and development of children with X and Y chromosome aneuploidy from infancy to pubertal age: The Toronto study. *Birth Defects: Original Article Series,* 1982, *18,* No. 4.

Stewart, D., Netley, C., Bailey, J., Haka-Ikse, K., Platt, J., Holland, W., & Cripps, M. Growth and development of children with X and Y chromosome aneuploidy: A prospective study. *Birth Defects: Original Article Series,* 1979, *15,* 75–114.

Vandenberg, S., & Kuse, A. Spatial ability: A critical review of the sex-linked major gene hypothesis. In M. Witting & A. Petersen (Eds.), *Sex-related differences in cognitive functioning.* New York: Academic Press, 1979.

Waber, D. Sex differences in cognition: A function of maturation rate? *Science,* 1976, *192,* 572–574. (a)

Waber, D. Sex differences and rate of physical growth. *Developmental Psychology,* 1977, *13,* 29–38. (a)

Waber, D. Biological substrates of field dependence: Implications of the sex difference. *Psychological Bulletin,* 1977, *84,* 1076–1087. (b)

Waber, D. Neuropsychological aspects of Turner syndrome. *Developmental Medicine and Child Neurology,* 1979, *21,* 58–70.

Wada, J., Clarke, R., & Hamm, A. Cerebral hemispheric asymmetry in humans. *Archives of Nuerology,* 1975, *32,* 239–246.

Wagner, D. A. Memories of Morocco: The influence of age, schooling and environment in memory. *Cognitive Psychology,* 1978, *10,* 1–29.

Witelson, S. F. Sex and the single hemisphere: Specialization of the right hemisphere for spatial processing. *Science,* 1976, *193,* 423–427 (a).

Witelson, S. F. Early hemisphere specialization and interhemispheric plasticity: An empirical and theoretical review. In S. Segalowitz & F. Gruber (Eds.), *Language development and neurological theory.* New York: Academic Press, 1977.

Witelson, S. F., & Paillie, W. Left hemisphere specialization for language in the newborn: Neuroanatomical evidence of asymmetry. *Brain,* 1973, *96,* 641–646.

14

Recent Progress on
the Genetics of Stuttering[1]

KENNETH K. KIDD

INTRODUCTION

Stuttering is a relatively frequent disorder in the timing of speech, occurring among children and adults in almost all populations. It has long been known to "run in families" (Bloodstein, 1981; Kidd & Records, 1979; Van Riper, 1971). The observation that stuttering is familial immediately excites a geneticist. Given the high frequency of genetic polymorphism in man at the enzyme level (Harris, 1975) and at the DNA level (Wyman & White, 1980; Kan & Dozy, 1980; Panny et al., 1981; Bell, Karan, & Rutter, 1981), a familial concentration for any trait makes a strong prima facie case for, but of course is not proof of, genetic transmission. In other words, it seems likely that some of this tremendous genetic variation among individuals affects who will ever stutter and who will never stutter. Nonetheless, until recently, few people have ever seriously considered stuttering as even possibly attributable to genetic factors. Consequently, there have been very few studies of stuttering designed to investigate the possibility of genetic variation contributing to variation in susceptibility to stuttering.

The study that has been in progress at Yale for the past 8 years is the most extensive family study of stuttering ever undertaken. It is specifically designed to investigate genetic questions. The initial results of this study are now becoming available, but these new data do not completely elucidate the role of genetic factors in the etiology of stuttering. Even the existence of relevant genetic factors cannot yet be proved beyond all doubt. However, we now have a much

[1]This work has been supported in part by USPHS grants NS11786 and MH30929.

GENETIC ASPECTS OF
SPEECH AND LANGUAGE DISORDERS

clearer understanding of the multifaceted problem and some significant new findings have been made. These initial results will be briefly reviewed in this chapter. They illustrate the enormous difficulties in genetic studies of complex behavioral phenotypes. They also provide some clear directions for future research on stuttering.

THE YALE FAMILY STUDY OF STUTTERING

In the Yale study, information on nearly 600 stutterers and more than 2000 of their first-degree relatives was obtained. Approximately half of our data sample was collected by standardized interview of the proband (or in the case of a child, the proband's parent) and half by a self-report questionnaire covering the same material as the direct interview. The majority of the individuals invited to participate in the family study were diagnosed as stutterers by speech pathologists or trained clinicians, and were initially referred to us by the speech pathologist. Each referred stutterer became a potential proband in our study. We were concerned that every proband had a confirmed diagnosis of stuttering; however, we did not insist that the proband had ever been enrolled in therapy or currently stutter. We eliminated from the study all individuals with known mental retardation, epilepsy, cerebral palsy, or neurological disorders that might possibly be associated with a higher incidence of stuttering or suggestive of generalized neurological dysfunction. All probands who met the criteria were included in the study, without regard to family size or knowledge of stuttering in the family. Biased sampling of interesting families (those with the speech pathologist's prior knowledge of stuttering in the family) was a major concern to us; the seriousness of this problem was discussed with all clinicians involved in making the initial contacts.

Only families of European descent have been included in the analyses done so far. We made this restriction to eliminate a possible source of genetic heterogeneity, and also to minimize cultural differences.

Two definitions of stuttering were used—one for the proband and one for family members. First, stuttering in the proband was defined by the diagnosis from the speech pathologist. (A direct diagnosis by the interviewer was not always possible if the proband no longer stuttered or stuttered in only specific situations, or if the self-report form was used.) Probands with a questionable diagnosis of disfluency, or with other diagnoses such as cluttering or spastic dysphonia, were not included in the study. Although individual speech pathologists may have slightly different definitions of stuttering, their diagnoses were considered to be conservative and reliable.

Stuttering in other family members, if not diagnosed at some time by a speech pathologist, was defined as excessive repetitions or prolongations or "having trouble getting the word out." The information concerning disfluencies in first-degree relatives was obtained from the probands (or parents of the proband), and as all probands stuttered, they were all attuned to such speech disfluencies. A stutterer was always defined as one who had ever stuttered or ever stammered, which would include those who stuttered only as children. For such individuals we required a duration of at least 6 months to minimize confusion with normal developmental disfluencies. Any error in incidence figures introduced because of failure to directly interview all relatives is considered small and, if present, would only elevate the frequency of stuttering in the relatives.

THE NATURE OF STUTTERING

Definition of the Phenotype

An important aspect of any genetic study is a clear definition of the trait being studied. Van Riper (1971) defines stuttering as "a temporal disruption in the simultaneous and successive programming of muscular movements required to produce one of [a] word's integrated sounds [p. 404]." Most experts consider that stuttering is basically a disruption in the timing of speech, in the smooth flow of speech (Andrews & Harris, 1964; Bloodstein, 1981; Wingate, 1964). This disruption is characterized by the block which may be manifest as a repetition (usually of only part of a word), as a prolongation, or sometimes as a silent gap in the middle of a word (Soderberg, 1967; Van Riper, 1971). Wingate's (1964) diagnostic criteria include disruptions in fluency that are characterized by involuntary repetitions or prolongations of sounds or syllables and one-syllable words that occur frequently and that are not readily controllable. Wyke (1970) summarized four characteristics of stuttering: (a) most stutterers stutter on the initial sound of the word; (b) stuttering increases with the syllabic complexity of the word; (c) there is more stuttering with connected speech than with single words; (d) stuttering is reduced during singing, choral speaking, or the recitation of rhythmically accented verse and syllable-timed speech (e.g., talking in time with a metronome).

The criteria of these authors provide ample material for diagnosing a moderate to severe case. Difficulties arise in very mild or beginning cases, as with most disorders. Most normal young children are disfluent in some way. Johnson (1959) and his associates classified disfluencies in stuttering and nonstuttering adults and children into eight categories. They found that part-word repetitions and prolonged sounds were considerably more frequently exhibited by the stutteres whereas both groups exhibited revisions, incomplete phrases, and interjections. McClay and Osgood (1959) found that the repetitions in normal, "fluent" speech are 71% whole words, 17% phrases, and 12% part-word sounds. In stuttering speech the proportions are nearly reversed: 63% of the repetitions are part-word repetitions (Soderberg, 1967). Bloodstein (1960) similarly found part-word repetitions to be the single most common symptom in young stuttering children and progressively less common in older (ages 12–16) children. Bloodstein also found all of the other possible symptoms and the secondary concomitants to be present among young stutterers.

The concomitant behaviors of stuttering are many and extremely varied. Some stutterers have few observable concomitants and others have many; severe stutterers can develop a whole repertoire of these behaviors. Examples of such behaviors are eye blinks, head jerks, and facial grimaces. They tend to be automatically performed and are often unconscious. They are not part of the basic disorder but are believed to develop through a behavioral learning process involving various types of reinforcement. Overt concomitants often develop to distract attention away from the stuttering block but often remain as a habitual part of the stuttering behavior. Generally, these secondary behaviors are confined to the moment of stuttering and are not present while the stutterer is silent. Though they may be the most noticeable aspect of a particular stutterer's behavior, they are not primary components in diagnosis.

Differential diagnosis of stuttering involves distinguishing it from cluttering. Cluttering is a disorder of speech and language that is characterized by speech so rapid that whole syllables and words are omitted, resulting in essentially unintelligible utterances. Cluttering can be improved by telling the clutterer to slow down, to think about what he is saying. If the clutterer is speaking to a superior or is a little more anxious and concerned about his speech, the speech improves. In the same situations the speech of a stutterer may become worse. Unlike that of a stutterer, the speech of a clutterer is usually unaccompanied by fear, anticipation, any difficulty with specific sounds or words, or even an awareness of speaking abnormally. Thus, in terms of symptoms and reactions to situations, stuttering and cluttering are quite different. They also occur in different families. Cluttering can show autosomal dominant inheritance (Op't Hof & Uys, 1974); stuttering rarely shows such a simple pattern.

In summary, diagnosis of stuttering is not without difficulties. However, there is remarkable agreement of the important manifestations and a limited range of phenotypic expression. The relative simplicity of diagnosis in the majority of cases is exemplified by the accuracy with which laymen can identify stuttering (e.g., Howie, 1981). Though not used in this study, the findings that stutterers have abnormalities in their laryngeal movements even when the speech sounds fluent provides additional support for the distinctiveness of this disorder. Evidence strongly suggests that the fluent speech of stutterers frequently reveals features that are not found, to the same degree, in the speech of nonstutterers (Agnello, 1975; Zimmerman, 1980; Shapiro, 1980).

Relevant Characteristics of the Disorder

Age of Onset

Variable age of onset is one of those characteristics of stuttering that must be considered in both the design of a study and in the interpretation of data.

Onset is almost always in childhood. Data from Andrews and Harris (1964) and Morely (1957) can be used to calculate a cumulative risk distribution which shows nearly 50% of onsets by age 4, 80% by age 6, and 98% by age 10. Onset after the age of 12 is only rarely reported in the literature. In the rare cases of adolescent or adult onset, there is often evidence that it is actually a recurrence of childhood stuttering (Van Riper, 1971) or the onset can be traced to a specific organic or psychological problem (Manning & Shirkey, 1979). Young (1975) reviewed the literature on age of onset and concluded that "stuttering . . . has its onset in early childhood with essentially no new cases of any significant number after the age of nine [p. 51]." Compared to information available on prevalence and recovery, he considered the findings on onset to be "the most secure."

The onset distributions in our study (Seider, Gladstien & Kidd, 1983) are typical of those reported by others, but do differ in particulars from some. We find the earliest onsets occur with the onset of speech. The 50th percentile for onset is around age 4; the 90th percentile is reached by age 8, the 99th percentile by age 12. The range of ages at onset is from 1.5 years to 16 years with the exception of three reports of later onset—at ages 20, 21, and 43—among reports of onset for 437 stutterers. The mean age at onset is 5.2 years; the modal age at onset is 3 years. The distributions of ages at onset are similar for the two sexes except that the female recovered stutterers in the study have a significantly earlier mean age of onset.

Spontaneous Recovery

Recovery is a major phenomenon: A large proportion of stutterers recover before they become adults and have normal speech thereafter. The frequency of spontaneous recovery from stuttering has been reported to be as low as 36% (Cooper, 1972) and as high as 80% (Sheehan & Martyn, 1966). As different populations were used in different studies, it is difficult to compare studies or define a consensus frequency for recovery.

In our data we find that the sex of the stuttering relative definitely affects the rate of recovery among first-degree relatives of persistent adult stutterers: 66% of 68 female stutterers had recovered whereas only 45.5% of 91 male relatives had recovered (Seider, et al., 1983). Thus, among this completely ascertained group there is an appreciable rate of spontaneous recovery, but much less than the 80% rate often quoted. The rate of recovery might be different, possibly even higher, among randomly ascertained stutterers. In any case, the elevated risks of both recovered stuttering and of persistent stuttering among the relatives of persistent stutterers supports the common clinical conclusion that these are both variants of the same basic disorder and are not etiologically distinct.

Although we do not yet understand the factors determining why some stutters recover and other do not, it is generally agreed that individuals whose stuttering persists into adulthood are not likely to recover spontaneous fluent speech. Adult stutterers can learn to increase the frequency of fluent words spoken, but it is generally through a conscious mechanism of speech monitoring, not through the automatic system that nonstutterers use.

Sex Differences

Stuttering has a very marked sex effect. There is a well-documented preponderance of affected males over affected females. Van Riper (1971) reviewed 18 studies that report sex ratios among stutterers from two to one (males:females) up to five to one. This difference between the sexes appears to hold in all cultures and races. Interestingly, though noting the sex difference, most studies do not present prevalence data by sex. The study by Andrews and Harris (1964) is the only one that has followed a group entirely through the age of risk and hence reports a true lifetime prevalence, nearly 3%. Though they did not report this lifetime prevalence by sex, they did report the total number of children and the number of male stutterers and female stutterers. Assuming a 1:1 sex ratio in the population, the sex-specific prevalences are 4.5% for males and 1.9% for females. As pointed out by Ingham (1976), that study was not without its deficiencies. However, no comparable study exists. Our data confirm the sex effect (Kidd, Kidd, & Records, 1978), as will be discussed later.

Familial Concentration

Several studies have shown that the risk for stuttering among the relatives of a stutterer is markedly elevated above that of the general population or of normally speaking control groups (Wepman, 1939; Andrews & Harris, 1964; Kant & Ahuja, 1970). In the more than 20 pertinent studies compiled by Van Riper (1971), the proportion of stutterers with a family history of stuttering ranged between 24% and 80% with a median of 42%. With few exceptions, those studies did not attempt to state the number or frequency of affected relatives, or their relationship to the proband. Many of these studies used matched control groups; Andrews and Harris (1964) found a family history of stuttering for 38% of the stutterers but only 1.4% of the controls. Significantly, among 30 of the stutterers with a positive family history, 13 were reported to have had no direct contact with the stuttering relative, suggesting that in at least these cases, imitation or social learning probably did not play a major role in the etiology of the disorder. Of course, positive family history, even with a control group, conveys little useful information as it is a function of family size.

Wingate (1964) reported that 21% of males ($N = 32$) who had stuttered had relatives in their immediate families who also stuttered. The relatives who stuttered were all males. Of 18 female stutterers, 33% reported other stutterers in their immediate families, of whom 67% were males. Andrews and Harris (1964) also found that female probands have a higher frequency of affected relatives of both sexes than do male probands. Kay (1964) was the first to calculate risks for first-degree relatives by sex of proband and relative. Those data indicated significant differences for male and female relatives, a difference confirmed by our data (Kidd et al., 1978).

The frequencies of stutterers among the first-degree relatives of our adult stutterers are given in Table 14.1. Two major points are obvious: (a) the frequency of stuttering among males is greater than that among females and (b) the frequencies among relatives are higher than any estimates for the frequencies in the population in general. The male–female difference is highly significant statistically (Kidd et al., 1978; Kidd, Heimbuch, & Records, 1981). The increases over the population rates are difficult to test statistically because of the uncertainties in the sex-specific prevalences but the familial rates are sufficiently large that statistical tests are hardly important. Note that these risk figures are per individual relative; the frequency of families with a positive history of stuttering is even higher. Though less obvious to visual inspection, our data also confirm the finding in the data of Andrews and Harris (1964) that female stutterers have a higher frequency of affected relatives; the increase is statistically significant (Kidd et al., 1981).

Stuttering in Twins

Most early investigations of stuttering in twins were focused on the possibility of an increased prevalence of the disorder among twins as compared to singletons. The rate of stuttering reported among twin groups varies widely from 1.9% (Graf, 1955) to 20% (Nelson, Hunter, & Walter, 1945). Sampling deficiencies, lack of zygosity determinations, and failure to report the sex render most twin concordance studies of little value in quantifying familial frequencies. For example, Nelson et al. (1945) reported that 9 of 10 monozygotic (MZ) pairs and 2 of 30 dizygotic (DZ) pairs were concordant for stuttering. Although consistent with the frequencies reported by Andrews and Harris (1964) for siblings, these concordances are not sex-specific and hence provide little useful information.

Howie (1981) conducted a twin study of 30 same-sex twin pairs: 21 male

TABLE 14.1

Distribution of Stuttering among First-Degree Relatives of Adult Stutterers

	Male probands	Female probands
Fathers	54/294 = .184 ± .023	21/103 = .204 ± .040
Mothers	13/294 = .044 ± .012	12/103 = .117 ± .032
Brothers	71/366 = .194 ± .021	24/104 = .231 ± .041
Sisters	12/295 = .041 ± .012	17/133 = .128 ± .029
Sons	29/123 = .236 ± .038	19/53 = .358 ± .066
Daughters	11/122 = .090 ± .026	8/45 = .178 ± .057

pairs (12 MZ, 9 MZ) and 9 female pairs (5 MZ, 4 DZ). The diagnoses of zygosity for these twins were based on five criteria: blood typing, total finger ridge counts, maximal palmar ATD angle, cephalic index, and height. Pairwise concordance for stuttering was found to be significantly higher in MZ twins (58–63%, depending on diagnostic criteria for stuttering) than in DZ twins (13–19%). The more meaningful probandwise concordances were about 75% for both male and female MZ twins, but were only 45% for male DZ twins and 0% (all 4 pairs discordant) for female DZ twins. The interclass correlations of total disfluency scores were also significantly higher in MZ twins (.67) than DZ twins (−.09).

In an Italian population pairwise concordances for stuttering were 83% for MZ twins (12 pairs) and 10.5% for DZ twins (19 pairs) (Godai et al., 1976). Eight of the nine male MZ pairs were concordant and two of the three female MZ pairs were concordant. All nine male DZ pairs were discordant, one of the two female DZ pairs was concordant, and among the eight unlike-sex pairs, both stuttered in one, the male stuttered in four, and the female stuttered in three. Though these data give concordances that seem quite different numerically from Howie's, the numbers involved are quite small and the two studies are in broad general agreement. Both studies yielded results compatible with genetic hypotheses but these twin data, in themselves, shed little light on specific mechanisms of inheritance.

Etiologic Hypotheses

There have been many different hypotheses on the origin of stuttering. One that had a great deal of influence starting in the early 1940s and continuing through the early 1950s was the semantogenic hypothesis (Johnson & Associates, 1959). This hypothesis is based on the observation that all children normally have some difficulty with speech as they are learning to talk. According to Johnson, the negative reactions of parents and others in the child's environment to these disfluencies create the speech problem. Having been evaluated as a stutterer, the child began speaking differently in response to the parental pressure and anxieties and the help he received. Our data are not in agreement with such a hypothesis.

Van Riper (1971) has reviewed most of the many theories of stuttering and grouped them into three categories: (a) stuttering as a neurosis, (b) stuttering as a learned behavior, and (c) stuttering as an organic disorder. Van Riper (1971) considers that no theory in the first two categories adequately explains the origin of the initial disfluency, while no theory of an entirely organic nature can explain the development of concomitant behavior patterns that are such a major component of advanced stuttering. Bloodstein (1981) draws a distinction between theories about the nature of an individual block—the moment of stuttering—and theories about the onset of the disorder. He notes that, though separate, any theory about the onset must depend to some degree on the hypothesized nature of the block.

Bloodstein's (1981) theory of communicative failure was based on his study of 108 stuttering children. His viewpoint is that primary stuttering usually begins as a response of tension and fragmentation in speech. In the presence of communicative pressure, the speech of children who are subject to the threat of speech pressure becomes more tense and fragmented. Bloodstein noted that retarded language development, articulation errors, reading difficulty, cluttering, or any other communication problem may make children more or less susceptible to speech breakdown.

Virtually all theories about stuttering fail to account for the clear familial pattern. Even the social learning theories of stuttering (see, e.g., Bandura, 1969, pp. 318–328) do not account for the specific pattern, just for the possibility of nongenetic familial transmission.

We have found that (Seider, Gladstein, & Kidd, 1982) late-talking stutterers and their nonstuttering siblings had significantly more articulation problems than did the stutterers who were early or average talkers and their siblings. Thus time of language onset may be a fundamental problem that is related to subsequent development of speech difficulties. Another possibility is that for some individuals a primary problem of unknown etiology exists, and stuttering, late talking, and articulation difficulties are only different manifestations of this underlying problem.

Researchers regarding stuttering as a breakdown of speech function consider stuttering to be basically an organic disorder. Organic factors have been associated with stuttering since Aristotle, who speculated there was something wrong with the stutterer's tongue. The precise description of the organic abnormality has not clearly been identified. Interest in the larynx, neuromuscular organization, and cerebral dominance have been renewed.

Several theorists have asserted that some children may be predisposed to stutter by either genetic or constitutional causes. Recent theories suggest stuttering is a product of hereditary predisposition and environmental precipitating factors. These theories separate quite clearly the presence or absence of the basic problem (e.g., in timing of speech) from the severity of the stuttering and from any concommitant behaviors that may be present. This distinction is necessary because of the clear dependence of the symptoms at any specific time on the emotional and social context. If a stutterer is anxious or nervous, his stuttering is much worse; in a classroom his stuttering may be very severe but out with friends his stuttering may be almost nonexistent. Such short-term temporal variation is likely to be affected by contextual factors distinct from those affecting the persistence of stuttering into adulthood. Still other nongenetic factors may affect the concomitant behaviors.

Transmission Hypotheses

Cultural Transmission Hypotheses

The familial nature of stuttering has often been explained as the result of the attitudes and traits of parents also running in families (Gray, 1940; Johnson,

1959; Bandura, 1969). Such cultural transmission does not depend on the semantogenic hypothesis; other forms of parent–child interaction could very well be involved. Some of the characteristics of parents of stutterers that have been suggested by numerous investigators include the setting of high goals and standards of performance, high expectations and evaluations of speech, covert forms of parental rejection, maternal overprotection and oversupervision, with-holding of approval for accomplishments, an unwillingness to encourage inde-pendence, and submissiveness and low social dominance on the part of the parents. All such traits may be positively correlated between parent and child.

We have examined several cultural transmission hypotheses, either directly or indirectly, using our data and have consistently obtained negative results. The simplest model is one in which the behavior is mimicked—a child stutters because he mimics stuttering behavior in a parent. That hypothesis can be quite convincingly rejected because it cannot account for much of the transmission (Kidd et al., 1978). Of those probands who had a parent who stuttered, it was the father who stuttered in most cases; over half of the fathers who ever stut-tered had recovered before they became adults. Thus, in about 90% of all families neither parent stuttered at the time the proband was born so that no parental role model for stuttering existed. In total, only a very small percentage of all stutterers had any stuttering model they could mimic.

Several other analyses provide evidence against various cultural transmis-sion hypotheses. Several analyses of sibship patterns of 303 stutterers show nothing distinctive between the stuttering siblings and the nonstuttering siblings (Gladstein, Seider, & Kidd, 1981). These results argue against sibling mimicry being a factor in stuttering and exclude other hypotheses in which these non-genetic factors (birth rank, age separation, etc.) are postulated to modulate the occurrence of stuttering. Severity of stuttering in the proband, measured as frequency of disfluent words in a standard reading passage, also showed no correlation with frequency of "ever stuttered" in the relatives (Kidd, Oehlert, Heimbuch, Records, Webster, 1980).

As mentioned earlier, many hypotheses have been put forth about the behavioral traits of parents that might cause stuttering. Some of those traits might be culturally transmitted. In light of what is now known about the family pattern of stuttering, it is interesting to reevaluate some of those reports. Re-member that on average about 20% of the stutterers had a father who had at some time stuttered. In one study (Johnson, 1959) a question was asked about how often the parents corrected their child's pronunciation. A significantly greater proportion of mothers of stutterers responded "never" than did mothers of controls—about 25% of the mothers of stutterers versus 7% of the mothers of controls. This was interpreted as mothers of stutters being more permissive and having lower social dominance. The fathers displayed a similar trait, 21% versus 13% never corrected their child for pronunciation. Unfortunately, this study provided no information on whether or not those fathers (or mothers) who never corrected the child's speech had ever stuttered when they were children. If 21% of the fathers had themselves at some time been stutterers, might not they be expected to have different behavioral attitudes toward their child's stuttering? Knowing whether a parent ever stuttered is an important factor in understanding the behavioral attitudes. The psychosocial studies should be reevaluated as none of them has ever taken into account whether or not the parent being studied had ever stuttered.

Genetic Transmission Hypotheses

There are several reasons, a priori, for thinking stuttering might have a genetic component. First, completely apart from its familiality, which is well documented, stuttering is a specific speech disfluency that is distinct from other types of speech disfluency. A second reason for believing stuttering might be genetic is that one would expect genetic defects in speech. Speech is the newest, most uniquely human form of behavior. Higher primates seem to have the rudiments of language; chimpanzees; for example, have been taught to communicate with abstract symbols using a simple form of grammar (Bourne, 1977). However, chimpanzees do not have speech; only humans have speech. Speech is an extremely complex form of behavior. Speech production involves over 100 muscles. The muscular movements involved in going from the production of one sound to the production of the next are extremely complex and require a sophisticated servomechanism with complex feedback and monitoring. It is estimated that approximately 140,000 neuromuscular events per second are involved in the normal production of speech (Bateman, 1977). Thus, though humans are genetically difficult to study, the uniquely human nature of speech precludes an animal model specifically of stuttering.

Characterizing the Familial Pattern Stuttering does not show a simple pattern of inheritance in families. In some families only a parent stutters. In some families many relatives stutter. In some families nobody else among a large number of relatives has ever stuttered. Some families appear to show X-linked recessive inheritance of stuttering because a male stutterer will have an unaffected sister who has affected sons. However, families with an affected father and an affected son are found in sufficient numbers that X-linked inheritance is apparently excluded. The seemingly X-linked patterns can be attributed to the clearly sex-modified risks of stuttering: Males are more frequently affected than females, both among probands and among relatives.

Both the high familial concentration and the sex effect can be seen in Table 14.1, given earlier. The frequencies of relatives who have ever stuttered are not suggestive of any simple Mendelian pattern. Among the male relatives of male probands approximately 20% report having ever stuttered at some time in their lives, whether they had recovered before they became adults or still stuttered in adulthood. Among the female relatives, however, the frequency of having ever stuttered is much lower, on the order of 5–10%. Interestingly, among relatives of female probands, the same qualitative pattern exists, but the frequencies are

TABLE 14.2
Observed Percentages of Stuttering among Siblings

	Parental type	Brothers		Sisters	
		%	N	%	N
Male probands	N	18.0	300	1.8	226
	F	25.5	55	11.5	61
Female probands	N	17.8	73	9.5	95
	F	32.0	25	21.4	28

systematically higher. Statistically, the effect of sex on how frequently a relative stutters is highly significant. This sex difference in frequency of stuttering among relatives emphasizes that for stuttering the sex effect is a very real phenomenon and not the ascertainment bias of males more frequently seeking therapy (Kidd et al., 1978; Kidd et al., 1981).

Vertical Transmission One initial question to be asked of these data is whether vertical transmission exists: Does a parent stuttering increase the risk of an offspring stuttering? The presence of vertical transmission is a prerequisite to most genetic hypotheses. Our analysis divides the families into subsets. Families of adult probands were first classified by whether the proband was a male or a female. Both groups of families were then classified into four types according to stuttering in the proband's parents: (1) N, neither parent ever stuttered; (2) F, father ever stuttered; (3) M, mother ever stuttered; and (4) B, both parents ever stuttered. Table 14.2 gives the frequencies of stutterers among the brothers and sisters of the probands for the more frequent types of families. The frequency of stuttering increases markedly if the father of the proband also stuttered. Full logistic analysis of the entire multiway contingency table shows that this nonrandom distribution within families is statistically significant in a pattern that is a clear demonstration that stuttering shows both vertical transmission within families and sex-modified expression (Kidd et al., 1981).

These analyses do not assume a genetic hypothesis but simply demonstrate that if a parent also stuttered the risk to other siblings increases. That finding is not proof that the transmission must be genetic, but it does indicate that there is transmission through these families of something that is related to stuttering. Moreover, whatever is transmitted also interacts with the sex of the individual: It takes more of this transmitted susceptibility to make a female become a stutterer. Conversely, by starting with a female stutterer as a proband, one is selecting families with more of these transmitted factors and hence one finds a higher frequency among the proband's relatives.

Genetic Models As already discussed, we have found no cultural hypothesis to explain this transmission pattern. However, some genetic models can explain it. Though stuttering does not show a clear single-gene pattern, its pattern may be explained by one of the more general threshold models. The single-major-loucs (SML) model has three genotypes, each with sex-specific probabilities of being affected (Kidd & Spence, 1976). The probabilities arise by considering nongenetic variation to determine a liability distribution around each genotype mean. A sex-specific threshold then divides the distribution to determine who does and who does not stutter. Heterozygotes would stutter if they have a sufficiently stressful environment while homozygotes would not stutter if they have a sufficiently benign or ameliorating environment. The positions of the thresholds and the gene frequencies can be varied to find the best explanation of the data. Note that according to this model all of the transmission is genetic.

Results for the single-major-locus hypothesis applied to our data are given in Table 14.3. This solution explains the family data quite well. The gene frequency estimated is 4%—not a rare gene, but not a very common one either. Most individuals in the total population lack the gene. About 8% of the population is heterozygous and less than 2 in a 1000 are actually homozygous. The penetrances, the probabilities that individuals with particular genotypes will ever stutter, can be different for males and females. Both the male and female penetrances are virtually zero for homozygotes for the normal genotype; both are one (or 100%) for homozygotes for the stuttering allele. A striking sex difference is found for heterozygotes: Penetrance is about 40% for a heterozygous male but only 11% for a heterozygous female. These parameter values predict a lifetime prevalence of ever stuttering at some time in childhood of around 4% for males and around 1% for females, approximately the values reported.

Finding an acceptable solution does not constitute proof that a single locus is responsible for stuttering, but it is highly suggestive. Especially noteworthy is that the model does not require that the interaction of genetic and nongenetic factors be confined to heterozygotes and yet biological principles would suggest that interaction is most likely to be significant in heterozygotes.

Any initial confidence in the applicability of the SML model to stuttering is weakened by the finding that other quite different genetic models can also explain the observed familial pattern (Kidd et al., 1978; Kidd, 1980). Thus, the

TABLE 14.3
Single-Major-Locus Analysis of Stuttering—Estimates of Genetic Parameters

	Genotypes		
	NN	NS	SS
Male penetrances	.005	.378 ± .025	1.0
Female penetrances	<.001	.107 ± .019	1.0
q = frequency of S = .040 ± .007			

TABLE 14.4

Recovered and Persistent Stutterers among Relatives of Adult Persistent Probands (Frequencies Show Significant Heterogeneity)[a]

Relationship to proband	Relatives of male probands			Relatives of female probands		
	Total ever stuttered	Number recovered	Percentage recovered	Total ever stuttered	Number recovered	Percentage recovered
Fathers	46	25	54	19	10	53
Mothers	13	9	69	12	10	83
Brothers	60	16	27	23	11	48
Sisters	10	6	60	14	5	36

[a]Data from Seider et al., 1983.

findings are encouraging for genetic hypotheses in general but the questions of exactly how susceptibility to stuttering is determined and transmitted are left unanswered.

Though severity of symptoms by one measure appears unrelated to transmission of stuttering (as discussed earlier), *severity* defined in some other way might be correlated with susceptibility and help resolve the uncertainty over the correct genetic model. An obvious candidate is persistence versus recovery. The breakdown of ever-stuttered relatives in our study according to recovery is given in Table 14.4. Analyses of these and additional data (Seider *et al.*, 1983) show that the pattern of recovery versus persistence among relatives is not consistent with persistent stuttering being a more severe form, either in general models of transmission or in various genetic models (Cox & Kidd, 1983). The data show persistent probands have an excess of persistent same-sex siblings. This may be the result of nongenetic factors affecting recovery or may be attributable to an ascertainment bias of some sort. Additional work on this question is clearly indicated.

FUTURE DIRECTIONS

We are not yet able to conclude what causes stuttering, but we can more clearly state the questions that need to be answered. Such questions include the following:

1. Can other statistical analyses yield more specific answers as to possible genetic mechanisms?
2. Why are females more resistant to the transmitted factors for susceptibility to stuttering?
3. Why do some stutterers recover and other persist?
4. Can the underlying transmitted susceptibility state be detected or revealed by some test?

5. Is there any way to prove that the susceptibility is genetic? We are now in the process of examining some of those questions.

As discussed by Pauls in Chapter 9 of this book, there are other statistical approaches to genetic analyses that are more powerful than those used so far on the available data. Some of those, such as PAP (Hasstedt & Cartwright, 1979), are being applied to the existing data. However, those methods seem to be most powerful with large, multigenerational pedigrees whereas our data are most complete and accurate for only the first-degree relatives of our probands. Partly for this reason and partly to provide data for some of the other questions, we are now collecting additional data on a few extended families selected because they contain several stutterers and/or recovered stutterers. Each individual in these families is being studied quite extensively using personal interview, self-report forms, psychological tests, and psychophysiological tests such as a dichotic listening task. Genetic markers for linkage analyses are also being studied on these families in the hope of detecting a major locus affecting susceptibility to stuttering. We feel that this high-density-family paradigm will be especially useful for further understanding the enigma of stuttering.

ACKNOWLEDGMENTS

The work reported here is the product of the efforts of many people who have worked on this project in data collection and analysis: N. J. Cox, K. Gladstien, P. Hartigan, R. C. Heimbuch, J. R. Kidd, M. A., Records, and R. A. Seider. The final version of the chapter benefitted greatly from discussions with the workshop participants.

REFERENCES

Agnello, J. G. Voice onset and voice termination features of stutterers. In L. M. Webster & L. C. Furst (Eds.), *Vocal tract dynamics and dysfluency.* New York: Speech and Hearing Institute, 1975.

Andrews, G., & Harris, M. M. *The syndrome of stuttering* (Clinics in Developmental Medicine, No. 17). London: Spastics Society Medical Education and Information Unit in association with William Heinemann Medical Books, 1964.

Bandura, A. *Principles of behavior modification.* New York: Holt, Rinehart and Winston, 1969.

Bateman, H. E. *A clinical approach to speech anatomy and physiology.* Springfield, Ill.: Charles C Thomas, 1977.

Bell, G. I., Karam, J. H., & Rutter, W. J. Polymorphic DNA region adjacent to the 5′ end of the human insulin gene. *Proceedings of the National Academy of Sciences,* U.S.A. 1981, *78,* 5759–5763.

Bloodstein, O. Development of stuttering, I & II. *Journal of Speech and Hearing Disorders,* 1960, *25,* pp. 219–237, 366–376.

Bloodstein, O. *A handbook on stuttering.* Chicago: National Easter Seal Society for Crippled Children and Adults, 1981.

Bourne, G. H. *Progress in ape research.* New York: Academic Press, 1977.

Cooper, E. B. Recovery from stuttering in a junior and senior high school population. *Journal of Speech and Hearing Research,* 1972, *15,* 632–638.

Cox, N. J., & Kidd, K. K. Can recovery from stuttering be considered a genetically milder subtype of stuttering? *Behavior Genetics,* 1983, *13,* 129–139.

Gladstien, K. L., Seider, R. A., & Kidd, K. K. Analysis of the sibship patterns of stutterers. *Journal of Speech and Hearing Research,* 1981, *24,* 460–462.

Godai, U., Tatarelli, R., & Bonanni, G., Stuttering and tics in twins. *Acta Geneticae Medicae et Gomellologiae,* 1976, *25,* 369–375.

Graf, O. I. Incidence of stuttering among twins. In W. Johnson (Ed.), *Stuttering in children and adults.* Minneapolis: University of Minnesota Press, 1955.

Gray, M. The X family: A clinical and laboratory study of a "stuttering" family. *Journal of Speech and Hearing Disorders,* 1940, *5,* 343–348.

Harris, H. *The principles of human biochemical genetics.* Amsterdam: North-Holland, 1975.

Hasstedt, S., & Cartwright, P. Pedigree analysis package (PAP) (Technical Report, No. 13). Salt Lake City: Department of Medical Biophysics and Computing LDS Hospital and University of Utah.

Howie, P. M. A twin investigation of the etiology of stuttering. *Journal of Speech and Hearing Research,* 1981, *24,* 317–321.

Ingham, R. J. Onset, prevalence, and recovery from stuttering: A reassessment of findings from the Andrews and Harris study. *Journal of Speech and Hearing Disorders,* 1976, *51,* 277–283.

Johnson, W., & Associates. *The onset of stuttering: Research findings and implications.* Minneapolis: University of MInnesota Press, 1959.

Kan, Y. W., & Dozy, A. M. Evolution of the hemoglobin S and C genes in world populations. *Science* 1980, *209,* 388–391.

Kant, K., & Ahuja, Y. R. Inheritance of stuttering. *Acta medica auxologica,* 1970, *2,* 179–191.

Kay, D. W. K. The genetics of stuttering. In G. Andrews & M. M. Harris (Eds.), *The syndrome of stuttering,* London: William Heinemann Books, 1964.

Kidd, K. K. Genetic models of stuttering. *Journal of Fluency Disorders,* 1980, *5,* 187–201.

Kidd, K. K. Heimbuch, R. C., & Records, M. A. Vertical transmission of susceptibility to stuttering with sex-modified expression. *Proceedings of the National Academy of Sciences,* 1981, *78,* 606–610.

Kidd, K. K., Kidd, J. R., & Records, M. A. The possible causes of the sex ratio in stuttering and its implications. *Journal of Fluency Disorders,* 1978, *3,* 13–23.

Kidd, K. K., Oehlert, G., Heimbuch, R. C., Records, M. A., Webster, R. L., Familial stuttering patterns are not related to one measure of severity. *Journal of Speech and Hearing Research,* 1980, *23,* 539–545.

Kidd, K. K., & Records, M. A. Genetic methodologies for the study of speech. In X. O. Breakefield (Ed.), *Neurogenetics: Genetic approaches to the nervous system.* New York: Elsevier North-Holland, 1979.

Kidd, K. K., & Spence, M. A. Genetic analyses of pyloric stenosis suggesting a specific maternal effect. *Journal of Medical Genetics,* 1976, *13,* 290–294.

Manning, W. H., & Shirkey, E. A. Fluency and the aging process. In D. S. Beasley & G. A. Davis (Eds.), *Speech, Language, and Hearing: The Aging Process,* New York: Grune & Stratton, 1979.

McClay, H., & Osgood, E. I. Hesitation phenomena in spontaneous English speech. *Word,* 1959, *15,* 19–44.

Morley, M. *The development and disorders of speech in childhood.* Edinburgh: Livingstone, 1957.

Nelson, S. F., Hunter, N., & Walter, M. Stuttering in twin types. *Journal of Speech Disorders,* 1945, *10,* 335–343.

Op't Hof, J., & Uys, I. C. A clinical delineation of tachyphemia (cluttering): A case of dominant inheritance. *South African Journal of Medical Sciences,* 1974, *48,* 1624–1628.

Panny, S. R., Scott, A. F., Smith, K. D., Philips III, J. A., Kazazian, H. H. Jr., Talbot, C. C. Jr., & Boehm, C. D. Population heterogeneity of the Hpa I restriction site associated with the β-globin gene: Implications for prenatal diagnosis. *American Journal of Human Genetics,* 1981, *33,* 25–35.

Seider, R. A., Gladstien, K. L., & Kidd, K. K. Language onset and concomitant speech and language problems in subgroups of stutterers and their siblings. *Journal of Speech and Hearing Research,* 1982, *25,* 482–486.

Seider, R. A., Gladstien, K. L., & Kidd, K. K. Recovery and persistence of stuttering among relatives of stutterers. *Journal of Speech and Hearing Disorders,* in press, 1983.

Shapiro, A. I. An electromyographic analysis of the fluent and dysfluent utterances of several types of stutterers. *Journal of Fluency Disorders,* 1980, *5,* 203.

Sheehan, J. G., & Martyn, M. M. Spontaneous recovery from stuttering. *Journal of Speech and Hearing Research,* 1966, *9,* 121–135.

Soderberg, G. A. Linguistic factors in stuttering. *Journal of Speech and Hearing Research,* 1967, *10,* 801–810.

Van Riper, C. *The nature of stuttering.* Englewood Cliffs, N.J.: Prentice-Hall; 1971.

Wepman, J. M. Familial incidence in stammering. *Journal of Speech Disorders,* 1939, *4,* 199–204.

Wingate, M. E. Recovery from stuttering. *Journal of Speech and Hearing Disorders,* 1964, *29,* 312–321.

Wyke, B. Neurological mechanisms in stammering: An hypothesis. *British Journal of Disorders of Communication,* 1970, *5,* 6–15.

Wyman, A. R., & White, R. A highly polymorphic locus in human DNA. *Proceedings of the National Academy of Sciences, U.S.A.,* 1980, *77,* 6754–6758.

Young, M. A. Onset, prevalence, and recovery from stuttering. *Journal of Speech and Hearing Disorders,* 1975, *40,* 49–58.

Zimmerman, G. Articulatory behaviors associated with stuttering: A cinefluorographic analysis. *Journal of Speech and Hearing Research,* 1980, *23,* 108–121.

Glossary

allele: one of two, or more, variants of a gene with the same locus on a specified chromosome.

aneuploid: possessing a diploid number of chromosomes that is a near, but not exact, multiple (e.g., 45 or 47) of the haploid number of chromosomes (i.e., 23).

assertive or assortative mating: nonrandom selection of a mate, based on phenotypic or genotypic characteristics.

autosome: any chromosome with the exception of X and Y, the sex chromosomes.

chromosome: nucleoprotein bodies that normally are constant in number in humans (i.e., 46) and carry the genes.

concordance: in reference to twins, the situation in which both individuals exhibit a particular trait or disease. See also "discordance."

diploid: possessing two identical sets of chromosomes, excluding the sex chromosome in males. In humans, the diploid number is normally 46. See also "euploid."

discordance: in reference to twins, the situation in which only one twin exhibits a particular trait or disease. See also "concordance."

dizygotic (DZ): in reference to twins, resulting from fertilization of different ova by different spermatozoa. Also termed "fraternal" twins.

DNA: deoxyribonucleic acid, the genetic material, the chemical compound of which genes are made. Found in the cell nucleus from which it determines life functions.

dominance/dominant: capacity of an allele for phenotypic expression of a trait, when paired with a different allele that is not, or is only partly, expressed. See also "recessivity/recessive."

DZ: see "dizygotic."

euploid: possessing an exact multiple of the haploid number of chromosomes (e.g., in humans, 46). See also "diploid."

expressivity: described in terms of quality or quantity, the degree to which a particular trait is manifested.

familial: the occurrence of a trait or disease in at least two members of an immediate or extended family.

fraternal twins: see "dizygotic."

gamete: the mature reproductive cells of the female (ova) and male (spermatozoa). Also termed "germ cell."

gene: comprised of DNA, the basic unit involved in the transmission of heritable traits, generally occupying specific loci on a chromosome.

gene map/genetic map: visual representation of the relative distances between and linear order of genes belonging to certain groups (i.e., genetic markers).

genome: the complete endowment of hereditary factors.

genotype: an individual's total genetic constitution, resulting from a particular combination of genes.

haploid: possessing a single set of chromosomes. In humans, the haploid number is normally 23, and is found only in the gametes.

heritability: expressed in terms of a percentage, that portion of the phenotypic variance in one generation of a population which is genetically determined.

heterozygous: having two different alleles at a particular locus of a chromosome.

homozogous: having identical alleles at a particular locus of a chromosome.

identical twins: see "monozygotic."

index case: the individual whose trait or disease identification was instrumental in the investigation and identification of the same in other family members. Also termed "proband" and "propositus."

karyotype: for each individual, the sum total of chromosomal characteristics, such as number, size, shape, and grouping within the nucleus.

linkage: the association of genes not having the same loci yet found on the same chromosome.

locus/loci: gene site on a chromosome.

meiosis: prior to the formation of the mature reproductive cell (gamete), the two successive divisions of the nuclear chromosome, in which the chromosomes divide once, and the cell body twice, thus resulting in the haploid number.

Mendelian patterns of inheritance/Mendelian Laws: laws of heredity, first expressed by Gregor Mendel, which attempt to explain the manner in which genetic information passes between parent and progeny.

monozygotic (MZ): in reference to twins, resulting from fertilization of a single ovum; also termed "identical" twins.

mosaic: individual with adjacent but genetically different tissue types.

multifactorial inheritance: see "polygenic inheritance."

mutant: exhibiting mutation.

mutation: an alteration in the expected or established characteristics of an individual, as the result of changes in the genotype.

MZ: see "monozygotic."

pedigree: diagram depicting the geneological history of a family, illustrating the occurrence of a particular trait or disease in the members.

penetrance: expressed in terms of percentage, the number of individuals with a particular genotype who exhibit the trait phenotypically.

phenotype: the visible behaviors or traits that characterize an individual, resulting from the interaction of genotypic and environmental factors. See also "genotype."

polygenic inheritance: a type of genetic transmission in which numerous genes with varying loci are related to the manifestation of a particular trait.

polymorphism: the coexistence in a population of two or more alleles with a frequency too elevated to be considered a new mutation.

prevalance: within a particular population, the current number of cases of a trait or disease.

proband: see "index case."

propositus: see "index case."

recessivity/recessive: the inability of an allele to express a trait phenotypically, when paired with a different allele that is expressed, or dominant. See also "dominance/dominant."

recombination: process whereby new combinations of genetic material occur, resulting in offspring with different gene combinations than their parents.

sex chromosomes: the X and Y chromosomes, which are related to sex determination at fertilization.

sex-limited: a genetic characteristic found only in one sex, or having a reduced occurrence in one sex.

sex-linked: with reference to genes located on the X chromosome, and to traits (manifested in either sex) related to such genes. Also termed "X-linked."

X chromosome: one of the two sex chromosomes, found in both females and males.

X-linked: see "sex-linked."

Y chromosome: one of the two sex chromosomes, found only in males.

zygosity: related to the number of zygotes from which a multiple birth has resulted. See "monozygotic," "dizygotic."

SUBJECT INDEX

A

Adoption
  designs, 121–138
  studies, 15, 131–135
Animal models, 16–17, 28–30, 81
Aphasia, 60–61, 76–77
Articulation, *see* Delayed speech and language;
  Speech and language development
Autism, 3–4, 10–11, 27, 97

B

Blood flow technique, *see* Cerebral blood flow
  technique
Brain functioning, *see also* Cerebral blood
  flow technique; Cerebral lateralization;
  Dyslexia; Electrophysiological indicators
  of brain activity
  development, 81, 188–189
  localization
    of language areas, 76–77, 57–61
    by metabolic indicators, 53–69

C

Cerebral blood flow technique, 53–69
Cerebral lateralization, 90–96
Chromosomal analysis
  in autism, 10
  in delayed speech and language, 5
  in dyslexia, 8, 169–178
Cluttering, 7, 200
Cognitive development, 51, 131–134,
  179–195, *see also* Speech and language development
  sex chromosome aberrations, 179–195
  sex differences, 87–90, 185
Cognitive disorders, *see* Cognitive
  development

D

Delayed speech and language, *see also* Dyslexia; Genetic research; Language
  acquisition
  articulation impairment, 6–7, 46, 47–48, 50
  assessment, 13–14, 37–38, 43
  attentional deficits, 66–68
  characteristics, 37–52
  cognitive abilities, 51, 179–195
  definition, 12–15, 51
  environmental factors, 15–16
  etiology, 3–5, 11, 15, 41–42, 71–84, 101,
  139
  family studies, 4–5, 15, 51
  identification, 12–15, 37–38, 44, 46–48,
  50–51, 63–65
  karyotypes, 5–6